Katie Coutts'
Good Health –
THE ALTERNATIVE WAY

KATIE COUTTS'
GOOD HEALTH – THE ALTERNATIVE WAY

Katie Coutts
WITH Marion Quinn

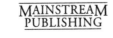

MAINSTREAM
PUBLISHING

EDINBURGH AND LONDON

First published in Great Britain in 2001 by
MAINSTREAM PUBLISHING COMPANY (EDINBURGH) LTD
7 Albany Street
Edinburgh EH1 3UG

ISBN 1 84018 419 1

A catalogue record for this book is available from the British Library

Typeset in Florentine, Garamond and Gill
Printed and bound in Great Britain by
Creative Print and Design Wales

Contents

Introduction

For as long as I can remember, I have been interested in ancient alternative medicine. I'm by no means a historian – in fact, history was my worst subject at school – but the history of medicine, be it conventional or unconventional, has always fascinated me. For centuries people have used plants, herbs and other natural produce as medicine, usually very successfully. I find it quite sad in a way that just because someone in more recent times discovered penicillin and other medicines, which today we class as 'conventional or normal', ancient remedies have been pushed to one side.

Having said that, over the years and definitely in the last five years, I have noticed the trend begin to turn again – this time in favour of ancient medicine. I'm by no means against conventional medicine, but I do find it interesting that we have so much more confidence in today's medicine, which is in fact very young, than we have in remedies which have been around for thousands of years. Don't get me wrong. Man has certainly come very far in finding cures for this and that. But I believe the human body these days suffers from a great many more illnesses than it did in the days before the advent of what we now call accustomed medicine.

To this effect I have personally carried out survey after survey – mainly for my own curiosity, I must add – whereby I ask my clients what their opinion is on normal, or prescriptive, medicine. The replies have been pretty similar. Most of us would rather try out medicines prescribed to us by our GPs than use alternative medicine as a first resort. There is, however, some contradiction: I've also discovered during these surveys that a great many people are aware of the sometimes ghastly side effects caused by today's medicine. The majority of my clients come to me *after* conventional medicine has failed to help the problem.

Alternative medicine is, like everything else, a personal belief, and more and more people are beginning to have greater faith in our old ways. With this in mind, Marion Quinn and I have aimed to compile a comprehensive yet lighthearted look at how best the general public can appreciate and use alternative medicine – an accessible, easy-to-follow reference book which readers can have at hand, rather like a dictionary, so that they can act quickly as soon as an ailment or illness begins. There are already dozens of books on the subject, but they tend to range from the beautifully illustrated to the quite impossible to comprehend. In many of them, the text is highly intellectual and basically way above the average person's head. We believe that the average person in the street has a right to know about, and to understand, alternative medicine.

I personally do not have any qualifications – at least not on paper – pertaining to either alternative or normal medicine. I don't expect those with qualifications to endorse this book, nor do I even expect them to read it, but there are very few of us who have letters after our names or who have vast scientific knowledge. What I can say is that I have studied alternative medicine for almost ten years and have practised it for seven years. With Marion, my ultimate aim is to highlight the benefits of alternative medicine as clearly as possible to the average reader – layperson to layperson.

Katie Coutts
March 2001

A-Z of Ailments

Abscesses

Everyone develops skin infections at some time in their life. If you have a cut that becomes red or swollen, starts oozing fluid and is really painful, then yours has become infected and is almost certainly what is known as an abscess. If it is deep-rooted, then the chances are that the area around it will also become swollen.

There are certain herbs that are very effective in treating minor abscesses, and the emphasis is on minor. Always remember that if it is seriously infected, or becomes worse, then you should see a doctor, so don't mess about. I don't want any limbs falling off! Seriously, alternative medicine is there to be used sensibly and hopefully it will help. If in doubt, always consult a doctor.

TEA TREE OIL: I personally use tea tree oil all the time as an antiseptic. Its many qualities are good against bacteria, although I would add that people who are sensitive to it might find it irritates the skin. You could try either bathing the affected area in diluted oil or soak some on a cloth to place over the abscess. Just don't try taking tea tree oil, even a small quantity can be poisonous. (See Tea tree oil, page 233.)

CALENDULA: Like tea tree, calendula reduces inflammation and promotes healing. Pour a cup of boiling water over a teaspoonful of dry petals. Then soak a cloth in the liquid and apply as a compress. Calendula also comes in many creams. Ask at your health food store. (See Calendula, page 144.)

COMFREY: Comfrey's healing agents may well help heal an abscess.

Again, you can find skincare products containing comfrey in many health stores. (See Comfrey, page 154.)

GARLIC: Applying garlic to the skin can cause irritation in some people. If you're not one of them, you can try putting a teaspoonful of garlic powder in a cup of hot water, then soak a cloth in it. Apply the cloth to the affected area. Alternatively, you can cut a clove open and tape it on.

ECHINACEA: This is one of my favourites for lots of things. Taken as a tea it can boost the immune system generally, so if you have an infected cut, try drinking some. (See Echinacea, page 154.)

Acne

Just think, if I had the cure for acne I'd be rich. Acne is such an annoying thing to have, the scourge of adolescence, the thing that all teenagers dread getting, and so hard to get rid of, if the amount of people at skin clinics is anything to go by. There are prescription drugs that can help but many have controversial side effects. As if teenagers weren't moody and depressed enough, I hear you say. I can't make extravagant promises, I'm afraid. But natural remedies are often the safest way to help your skin. This is what I suggest.

PREVENTION: This is so difficult. Unfortunately everyone's skin type is different. Some teenagers don't even get one spot. While others, eating the same food, using the same soap, can be covered. Sometimes persistent long-term acne is caused by a hormonal imbalance, so it's important this is checked out first. Correcting the balance can be a cure in itself. If your teenage son or daughter has acne, be kind, understanding and helpful. Don't dismiss the problem, or make negative comments. It won't cure it but it will help them feel better about themselves. Encourage them to clean their skin carefully and regularly, often patting it with hot water to open the pores and dabbing it gently dry. Picking and squeezing the spots makes it worse, and rubbing spreads the infection round the face. Changes in diet can help. Fatty and sweet foods in particular should be avoided, or cut down. Eating plenty of greens is good for acne, as is drinking lots of water to keep the system flushed and the skin moist. Daily vitamin supplements of vitamins A, B complex and C can also help, as can mineral supplements such as zinc. And let's not forget the sunshine. Maybe it's the vitamin D, maybe it's just that it helps the spots to dry out, but it certainly does no harm to be out getting some sun when it's there.

CAMOMILE: I find this useful for reducing the grease content on the skin and helping the spots heal quicker, without leaving scars. Just boil up some camomile tea and when it has cooled a little, dab it on carefully, holding it on each spot for a moment or so. Doing this once a day is a little time-consuming but if it helps then it's worth it. While it doesn't clear the spots completely, it certainly helps keep the skin looking fresh and clean. (See Camomile, page 145.)

BURDOCK: Like camomile, this is a good cleanser, although initially it can make the problem worse. That's because of what it's bringing out of the skin. Although you can make your own infusion, with a problem like acne, that's unfortunately not going to go away overnight, you might be better off buying supplements. It's much less time-consuming and that's coming from one who just loves boiling up things! The root is more powerful here than the leaf. (See Burdock, page 140.)

EVENING PRIMROSE OIL: In some instances taking capsules of evening primrose oil has helped, especially where hormonal things are concerned. Always worth a try. (See Evening primrose oil, page 165.)

DANDELION: This is a herb known for it's detoxifying qualities. Obviously with acne the body is getting rid of a lot of unwanted toxins through the skin, so this might help, if taken as a tea. (See Dandelion, page 159.)

GARLIC: Garlic is good for healing many other skin conditions, so I'd give it a shot here, probably in capsule form. (See Garlic, page 174.)

RED CLOVER: This is one that probably grows in your garden. Try boiling up the flowers in water, till a third of the water has boiled away, straining and applying to the spots. If you don't boil too much, you can keep the mixture in the fridge for three days.

CALENDULA: Calendula cream might also help if applied to the spots. (See Calendula, page 144.)

WITCH HAZEL: I don't think witch hazel on its own can cure acne, but adding a teaspoon to some of the above external skin washes, can't do any harm. (See Witch hazel, page 252.)

PINEAPPLE: Generally pineapple is very good for the skin. So much so that it's increasingly found as an ingredient in beauty products. As well as eating lots, you could try cutting up a raw pineapple and placing it on your face for 15 minutes as a regular treatment.

A WORD OF CAUTION: Please refer to the instructions for the individual remedy and remember not to take anything that is meant for external use.

INTERESTING FACT: The Victorians used sulphur to treat acne.

Altitude sickness

Although this is called altitude sickness, unlike motion sickness, there is sometimes very little vomiting involved. The symptoms are headache, dizziness, heart palpitations, tiredness, thirst, shortness of breath and nausea. It does not have anything to do with the change in altitude, but the thinning of oxygen that occurs at higher levels. Mountain climbers, therefore, are most at risk of suffering from it. Air travellers are protected when the little masks drop down. But it can lead to all sorts of other problems in a climbing situation, as well as making you unwell during or after a climb. So it is helpful to know what you can do to prevent it.

PREVENTION: Knowing that if you don't climb, you won't get it, isn't really the sort of advice you want here. Slow ascents always give the body time to adjust. The real problem comes when you are taking part in a rapid ascent. Since the change in oxygen level causes thirst, which in turn leads to dizziness and headaches, you can ward off some of these effects by drinking plenty before you start and while you are on your way through the climb. By drinking I mean drinking water. Alcohol just makes things worse! Soups are always good because they are a foodstuff as well as a drink and you can put some of the herbs and vegetables in them that help increase the blood flow to the brain. Garlic, onions, carrots, parsley, tomatoes and dill are some of those. Some of the herb teas, which help prevent headache and fatigue generally, might be good too (see Headache, page 165). Just stay off the sleepy relaxing ones like camomile. Not a good idea in a climbing situation!

GINGKO BILOBA: Because gingko increases the blood flow to the brain, it could probably help prevent you getting altitude sickness, if extracts are taken before and during your climb. (See Gingko biloba, page 177.)

GARLIC: Garlic helps thin the blood, keeping it flowing well, so taking capsules with you might be an idea if you're a climber. (See Garlic, page 174.)

A WORD OF CAUTION: Please refer to the references for the individual herbs for further advice and always take according to the manufacturer's instructions.

INTERESTING FACT: Most altitude sickness occurs at heights of over 7,000 feet.

Alzheimer's disease

Alzheimer's is the most common form of dementia – a progressive brain disease. Protein deposits develop throughout the brain. A further abnormality is the formation of twisted molecules. While no one can say for certain what triggers these processes, the results are all too well known. Memory loss, personality loss, ability loss. Loss of a loved one to a world we cannot reach. A lot of losses.

Until a few years ago there was no way to treat Alzheimer's and although some drugs are now available – and studies show they can bring about an improvement for some people – sadly, and invariably, the symptoms return.

Alzheimer's is fairly rare in the under-65 age group. It is reckoned, however, that one in five of us will have some degree of dementia by the time we're 80. So is there anything we can do? Well, to make sure that we're one of the safe four, we can try taking certain herbs and foods that boost the memory. Since scientists looking for a cure for Alzheimer's are also examining what these foods contain, they might also help slow the process of deterioration for sufferers.

BRAZIL NUTS: These contain a generous amount of lecithin, a substance that sharpens the brain. They are widely available and pleasant to eat.

DANDELION: Like Brazil nuts, dandelion flowers are a good source of lecithin. Dandelion can be taken in many forms. (See Dandelion, page 159.)

FAVA BEANS: So they've had a bit of a bad press recently, thanks to a certain doctor's eating habits, fava beans are nonetheless full of lecithin. Again, these are easily obtainable – visit your health food store – and if you don't want to wash them down with a nice Chianti, you can try putting them in soup.

ROSEMARY: If you're familiar with Shakespeare, you'll know the quote from Hamlet, 'There's rosemary, that's for remembrance.' Indeed rosemary has a long history as a memory-enhancing herb and perhaps is worth considering closely. It's easy to take – it comes in tea form, or it can be sprinkled on food. Also, since several of the compounds in it can be absorbed through the skin, the chances are some might cross the blood-brain barrier. So using a shampoo with rosemary in it, or adding rosemary tincture to your own herbal one, might well be worth a try.

GINGKO BILOBA: Studies have shown that gingko biloba improves circulation and is helpful with memory loss and ageing. (See Gingko biloba, page 177.)

INTERESTING FACT: Although Alzheimer's mainly affects people over the age of 65, the youngest known case is 28.

Anaemia

Basically, anaemia happens when there are low concentrations of the red pigment haemoglobin in the blood. These red cells are needed to take the oxygen round our bodies and if this doesn't happen then certain things, like muscles and our brain, can't function properly. The main symptoms are fainting, dizziness, paleness, breathlessness, palpitations, depression and profound exhaustion. But anaemia itself is a symptom of other conditions, one that needs to be identified. So if you suspect you have it, your first step should be to go to the doctor. There are three root causes: problems with the bone marrow; iron or vitamin deficiency, sometimes caused by the stomach not digesting the 'goodness' in food properly, even though you think you're taking the right things; and destruction of the blood cells by disease, immune disorders or excessive bleeding. This can be due to heavy periods, fibroids, or a bleeding stomach ulcer. It is therefore important that the underlying cause is discovered and treated so that this condition can be successfully managed. If you don't go to the doctor because you're worried, then you're just making things worse, risking your health, and indeed your life, if that kind of bleeding continues.

PREVENTION: Okay, so I'm sounding a bit heavy here! That's because it's a condition you can't ignore. Can you prevent it? Well, anaemia of the deficiency type often occurs in pregnant women and this is something that is generally discussed at antenatal appointments. Eating iron-rich foods can help. And these, in the main, are; fish, chicken, blackcurrants, fresh fruit, beetroot, wholemeal breads, green vegetables and lean meat. Orange juice is a good source of vitamin C, which can also help, and if you're really worried, then taking iron tablets does help. Anaemia caused by heavy periods – and often young teenage girls are at risk here – can also be helped, and perhaps prevented, by this diet and by taking iron supplements. Despite the fact that vegetarians eat mainly, well – vegetables – they are often at risk, because the iron they get from their diet is less absorbable.

Taking iron tablets can help, however, and the best way to wash them down is with orange juice. Both coffee and tea block iron absorption. So if you do have iron-deficiency anaemia then cut down on both.

DANDELION TEA: This is also a traditional remedy for anaemia, because of the vitamins it contains. Ask for it at your health shop. When you make it, add a spoonful of honey, which is also very good. (See Dandelion, page 159.)

NETTLE JUICE: Again, traditionally this has been used for hundreds of years to treat this condition. You can boil a handful of leaves in water. Remember to wear gloves when you pick them. Then allow to steep for 15 minutes, strain, then drink. (See Nettle, pages 207–8.)

KELP: Either sprinkle dried kelp on your food or take kelp tablets. Kelp was traditionally used to perk up the circulation. It's also very good as a digestive aid.

CAMOMILE: Rather than drinking ordinary tea, if you suffer from anaemia, I would recommend this instead. As well as helping you rest and improving your digestion it should also help boost the circulation and strengthen the blood. (See Camomile, pages 145–7.)

A WORD OF CAUTION: Please refer to the references for the individual remedies to find the one that is suitable and safe for you.

INTERESTING FACT: A hundred years ago physicians were mystified by a disease that they classed as anaemia, largely because the haemoglobin was somewhat low. There were many different symptoms, and these differed from patient to patient. The main ones were feelings of persistent weakness, irritability, loss of interest, inability to concentrate, depression and chronic fatigue to the extent that a sufferer could not move a muscle some days, yet was fine the next.

Angina

Angina is caused by a hardening or narrowing of the arteries and is a form of heart disease that causes chest pain. There are three types: stable, variable and unstable. The first can come on after exercise, the second during exercise, and the third can lead to a heart attack. Straight away I'm going to say that anyone experiencing new, severe chest pain or worsening of previously mild angina, must seek medical advice immediately. Anyone with angina should not only be seeing a doctor but should follow their recommendations. Other things can help and are outlined below.

LIFESTYLE: Developing any serious condition means changing your lifestyle, whether you like it or not. Stopping smoking, if you do so, is one of the most positive things you can do. Apart from the obvious health risk, by continuing to smoke you are reducing the effectiveness of whatever treatment you are receiving. Talk this over with your doctor first, but exercise, even just a daily ten-minute walk, can also help increase the heart blood flow significantly.

DIET: Cut out the coffee. It's bad news for angina sufferers. Remember my 'eat healthy, stay healthy' slogan. I swear by it and in many ways we are what we eat. Cut down on all the fatty foods, add more fruit, fruit juices and vegetables to your diet. If you like puddings, then start making them with fruit, which helps the heart. Try our heart soup (recipe on page 259) for a special dish. Being told to watch your diet doesn't mean eating a lot of boring things. It opens up wonderful opportunities for you to be creative with food and make your own dishes.

HAWTHORN: Hawthorn works by opening the arteries and decreasing cholesterol levels. (See Hawthorn, page 183.)

BILBERRY: If you're a sufferer or have a family history of heart disease, you can try adding bilberries to your diet on a regular basis. (See Bilberry, page 134.) Other fruits that might help are cherries, cranberries and raspberries. Just think of the wonderful fun you can have concocting dishes with these.

GINGER: As well as containing anti-cholesterol properties, ginger strengthens the heart muscle. Either take a teaspoon a day of powdered ginger, or start adding it to your cooking. Ginger and carrots is a wonderful way of eating both. (See Ginger, page 175, and the recipe on page 262.)

GARLIC: According to one study, eating one clove of garlic a day cuts cholesterol by 9 per cent. If you have heart problems, get plenty of garlic on your food. (See Garlic, page 174.) Never mind warding off the vampires, think about warding off heart disease as well!

ASPIRIN: Studies have shown that taking a low-dose aspirin a day can prevent a heart attack, and I know old ladies who swear by it. If you don't want to take a conventional aspirin, and I personally don't sniff at it, then try a herbal one. Ask at your health store for herbal aspirin or tea containing willow bark.

A WORD OF CAUTION: Everything we have mentioned is easily obtainable but please refer to the appropriate sections for use. Hawthorn in particular is a powerful herbal medicine, otherwise the rest are safe to use.

INTERESTING FACT: The Chinese use kudzu to treat angina. Kudzu can be grown but beware, similar to ivy, it spreads and it spreads and it spreads!

Arthritis

Arthritis means joint inflammation. Boiled down further there are actually many different diseases that produce joint inflammation and pain. The two most common, however, are osteoarthritis – where stiffness develops gradually in the hips, knees, spine, hands and feet – and rheumatoid arthritis – which causes crippling joint deformity and destroys the bones. Rheumatoid arthritis usually affects the hands, but can strike other joints as well. The symptoms include fatigue, fever, loss of appetite, as well as joint swelling, pain and warmth. Women tend to have it more than men.

PREVENTION: There is no easy way to prevent getting arthritis. It is often hereditary, so if your family is riddled, so to speak, and you're young enough to do something about it, then you can try taking remedies to keep the joints in good order. People doing very physical jobs and sportsmen and women are often at risk because of the amount of injuries they suffer. Since arthritis is sometimes associated with an excess of acid waste matter in the body, diet can certainly help. Cut down on red meat, cheeses, sugary foods, tea and coffee. If you're eating lots of foods that keep the acid from building up then the joints are going to be healthier, generally, whether you have arthritis already or are concerned about getting it. These foods include:

PINEAPPLE: One of the compounds helps prevent inflammation generally as well as getting rid of one of the substances that causes arthritis. Eating lots of it is certainly good advice.

OREGANO: This is a good antioxidant – helping the body get rid of the bad things. So get it on your food generally. (See Oregano, page 211.)

ROSEMARY: Has the same effect. (See Rosemary, page 226.)

CELERY: Eaten regularly, this is a good addition to a preventative diet. (See Celery, page 148.)

BROCCOLI: Some studies show that people who have arthritis are low on a compound that helps the body get rid of toxins. Broccoli, cabbage, potatoes, watermelon, oranges and peaches, all contain this compound. So eating generous amounts of these will certainly help.

GINGER: Now we're coming to those that help sufferers. Ginger is very good for relieving pain and swelling. In addition to sprinkling it onto your food, you can look for supplements or teas. (See Ginger, page 175.)

RED PEPPER (CAYENNE POWDER): This is one that goes in my food all the time. Not only does it contain pain-relieving qualities, it can also be effective if you rub it on the skin.

NETTLE: Look for a good nettle tea, or make your own. Nettle contains substances that help the bones retain calcium, thus keeping them healthy. (See Nettle, page 207.)

DEVIL'S CLAW: I personally recommend this strange sounding herb for arthritis and being a sufferer myself I know what I'm talking about! It flushes out the uric acid, which builds up on the joints, it's very good for reducing inflammation and keeping the tendons in good working order. It's also excellent for gout.

BURDOCK: This is another herb I feel has a number of good qualities and is so easy to take and come by these days. (See Burdock, page 140.)

A WORD OF CAUTION: Please refer to the individual reference for the remedy of your choice and follow all instructions properly. Remember, too, it takes time for herbals to work. Don't give up after one day because there's no miracle improvement.

INTERESTING FACT: Vitamin C has been shown to help stop osteoarthritis in guinea pigs.

Asthma

Asthma is on the increase and if you are a sufferer you know it is no joke. Asthma causes death. That's a simple fact. In extreme cases, perhaps, but nonetheless it's one that can be borne out by various facts and figures. Asthma is very much on the increase in Western civilisation, possibly because of growing pollution. No one can say for certain. If they could, perhaps we could do more about it. I don't know. What I do know is that if you, or any of your family, have asthma, you mustn't mess about. Follow your doctor's recommendations. They knows best. Asthma literally takes your breath away, so you must always be careful how you treat it.

PREVENTION: Because the actual cause is unknown, this is very difficult, so it makes more sense here to offer some advice about limiting attacks. I do believe that pollution has a lot to do with it, but as things stand there's not a lot you can do individually about that. Asthma is thought to be an allergy in some instances. So it's important, first of all, to determine if your attacks are being triggered perhaps by a foodstuff or cigarette smoke. Then there's chemical substances. Let's not pretend they're not everywhere, in your home, in your furnishings. Have you ever heard of 'Sick Building Syndrome'? Well, it's not the building that's sick. It's you. Ionised air, hot-air heating systems. Is any of this you? Because if it is, then maybe that's what's causing your problem? Stress also plays a role in asthma, as does severe anxiety. Stop a minute and look at your children, if they are sufferers. So much of their life often consists of what I call 'bundling'. And it's not 'bundling' as our forebears knew it. It's bundling into the car, bundling off to the childminders, bundling round to the shops, bundling off to the Brownies, the gym class, the riding lesson, to so-and-so's house, to every activity under the sun. We're all so busy bundling through our own lives and jobs, juggling the partner hoop, the children hoop, the housework hoop, the friends hoop, family life is often very fraught. Look for ways to de-stress yours if there is a sufferer in your family.

DIET: Tea, coffee, cocoa, chocolate and cola can all help asthma sufferers because they contain caffeine and other chemicals that help keep the bronchial tract open. So can eating foodstuffs that are high in vitamin C. If you try including lots of citrus fruits and strawberries in your diet, this should boost your levels (see Vitamin C, page 243). Other herbs and vegetables to include regularly in your diet are coriander, onion, cabbage, carrot, cranberry, sage, cayenne and fennel.

MAGNESIUM: Some studies show that people with asthma have low levels of magnesium. Either supplement this by taking tablets – many vitamins now come combined – or try to take more in your diet. (See Magnesium, page 148.)

VITAMIN B12: Again, the trace mineral in B12 helps the body deal with the substances that can trigger attacks.

LOBELIA: Lobelia capsules can help stop coughing spasms.

GINGKO BILOBA: This was used for thousands of years to treat coughs, allergies and asthma. It's also very easy to find. Try taking between 60 and 200 ml a day. (See Gingko biloba, page 177.)

LICORICE: Licorice tea can help soothe a sore throat and a cough, so might be helpful if you've got one. (See Licorice, page 195.)

MARSH MALLOW: The same goes for marsh mallow. (See Marsh mallow, page 200.)

A WORD OF CAUTION: Refer to the individual remedy and follow according to the instructions. Remember what I said at the start, the person who knows best is your doctor and I wouldn't recommend you messing about brewing licorice tea if you can't breath!

INTERESTING FACT: The Australians recommend stinging nettle. The extracts are easily available, or you can make a tea by boiling the roots and leaves with honey.

Bladder infections

Right away I'm going to say here that although men can, and do, develop bladder infections, this is mainly a women's thing. I could be really vulgar here and say why that is, but I'll refrain! But basically, because of this anatomical fact, the germs don't have so far to travel. Bladder infections are usually called cystitis and urinary tract infections, but it really doesn't matter what they're called – they're an absolute misery. A painful, burning sensation when you 'go' is bad enough. Especially when five minutes after you 'go', you need to 'go' again! In some cases, back pain, fever and blood tinged urine can develop. If it does, you must see a doctor. In fact, you really should be seeing a doctor full stop. Bladder infections are difficult to clear without an antibiotic and doing the 'herbal bit' doesn't mean you should suffer or be silly about it. What I'm doing here is looking at things that might help, especially if you suffer often. Most people who have a bladder infection will find that it's a reccurring fact of life! But the good news is there are things you can do to help.

PREVENTION: This doesn't mean you have poor hygiene, but it's worth stressing that a great many bladder infections are caused by the way people wipe themselves after going to the loo. Women in particular, obviously. It's a case of germs from the anal area – ones that live in the digestive tract – being swiped onto the urethra. Then they climb everywhere. I think you get the picture. Other people, too, find that they always get a bladder infection after being in a swimming pool or getting their feet wet. Obviously their system just doesn't like getting chills. So the answer to that one is simple. Sex, too, can bruise the urethra and cause infections. I can't very well say you know what to do there. Not indulging isn't much fun! Men who suffer bladder infections often have an enlarged prostate. There is a separate section on this (Prostate enlargement, page 94). Other good preventatives are to take lots of juice and foodstuffs that act as diuretics. That way any germs in the bladder are soon flushed out, never getting the chance to stay long enough and develop into anything nasty.

CRANBERRY JUICE: This is one of the best diuretics. But it also contains a substance that is largely antibiotic. You would have to drink a lot and it is rather high on calories. I am, however, a believer in the philosophy that every little helps and cranberry juice is good in a variety of ways. So start adding it to your diet every day. With some of these other remedies you just might kiss bladder infections goodbye! (See Cranberry, page 155.)

PARSLEY: Traditionally, this herb was used for bladder problems. It's easy to grow, so you can have a fresh supply, but it can also be bought dried and added to food. You can even try steeping the fresh herb and drinking the result. (See Parsley, page 213.)

ECHINACEA: This is a sort of herbal antibiotic especially when combined with goldenseal. It boosts the immune system fighting off infections. (See Echinacea, page 161.)

Breast-feeding

Okay, I have a confession to make. It's cards on the table time, and straightaway I'm going to say to you this is something I've never done. Nor do I think that makes me a bad mother. I'm an advocate of doing what I think and feel is best. I also think that too many women find themselves forced into doing something they're not happy with, which has repercussions for themselves and the new baby. No one should be pilloried or made to feel they're a failure when they've just done something very special. And they have! If, however, you are breast-feeding, and experiencing problems, there are certain simple herbs you can take that can help, so the special experience can continue.

PARSLEY (BREAST TENDERNESS, WEANING): Traditionally, women ate fresh parsley when they wanted to wean the infant, because it helps stop milk production. Parsley can also be used at this stage if your breasts are tender. Often this is caused by water retention and parsley is a diuretic. It's also very easy to buy from supermarkets. (See Parsley, page 213.)

JASMINE: Again, to suppress milk flow, apply fresh jasmine flowers to the breast. It's not clear why this works, but there are studies to prove that it does!

CALENDULA, LEMON JUICE, OLIVE OIL (SORE OR CRACKED NIPPLES): To prevent your nipples cracking or becoming sore, you can either rub on a little calendula ointment, obtainable from your health shop, or a mixture of lemon juice and olive oil. Also make sure that you wash and dry the breasts before and after feeding, as this can sometimes cause this condition.

ECHINACEA (CRACKED NIPPLES AND MASTITIS): Both sore, cracked nipples and mastitis, which is where the breasts become hard and very painful, can be soothed by taking a few drops of echinacea tincture three times a day. Echinacea is a herbal antibiotic, ideal for this kind of problem. (See Echinacea, page 161.)

DANDELION (MASTITIS): Boil a teaspoonful of chopped dandelion root in three cups of water, until half is boiled away. Then make a compress with the rest and apply to the breasts. Sounds funny? Well yes, but the Chinese have been doing it for hundreds of years.

MARSH MALLOW (MASTITIS, MILK FLOW): I think we have to take Mr Coles, a seventeenth-century physician, at his word when he says marsh mallow is for the 'paps of women, to procure a great flow of milk and assuage the hardening thereof'. I just hope it's the 'paps' and not the women he means to soften! Seriously, you can try making a salve by simmering mallow flowers in water and dabbing it on the breasts if they're sore and hard. Or ask at your health shop for products containing marsh mallow. It can also promote the milk flow. (See Marsh mallow, page 200.)

PEANUT (MILK FLOW): Yes, believe it or not, the humble peanut can promote milk flow. In China anyway! So if this is a problem for you, it's a very good and nutritious way to solve it. Unless you have an allergy of course, in which case try one of the other remedies. As you can see, there are quite a few.

GARLIC (MILK FLOW): There are studies that suggest eating a clove of garlic within an hour of starting to nurse, can be beneficial. Not only does it increase milk flow but for some reason it causes the babies to attach more readily to the breast. (See Garlic, page 174.)

FENNEL (MILK FLOW): Fennel has properties that are very similar to the female hormone oestrogen, and has been used for centuries to promote milk flow. Ask at your health shop for a drink containing it. Do not, however, take fennel oil, which is highly toxic. (See Fennel, page 167.)

RASPBERRY (MILK FLOW): Like fennel, raspberry has been used for hundreds of years to increase milk flow and it's quite a delicious way of doing it. You can choose to eat them fresh or try a raspberry tea, two or three times a day.

FENUGREEK (MILK FLOW): Ask at your health shop for products containing this herb. It contains compounds that have promoted breast milk flow since biblical times, believe it or not. I do. That's why I'm recommending it.

DAMIANA (MILK FLOW): This is excellent for many women's problems. If yours is that you can't produce enough milk, then perhaps you should give this one a go and, who knows, your cups might just overflow! (See Damiana, page 158.)

BLESSED THISTLE (MILK FLOW): Again, I wouldn't hesitate to recommend this herb for this problem. It's also very good for boosting the immune system, which is often a bit low at this time.

A WORD OF CAUTION: Please refer to the appropriate sections for the remedy you choose and remember to read the instructions on herbal supplements carefully. That said, these are all safe to use.

INTERESTING FACT: The idea of rubbing jasmine flowers on the breasts comes from India. In Britain they used to recommend goose dung! I think I know which one I prefer!

Bronchitis

Bronchitis, whether it's acute or chronic, is an inflammation of the trachea and the bronchial tract. It usually begins with a simple dry cough. In a matter of hours, however, that simple dry cough can become a hacking, mucus-producing nuisance that won't leave us alone. Fever can and usually does set in and, as with most respiratory infections, we feel weak. In fact, we feel awful. I think that's it in a nutshell, except to say that the elderly and people with weak immune systems are especially at risk of developing it if they have a respiratory infection and so should take care. Young children too. I think I spent the whole of my childhood with it. But that was no doubt down to a combination of damp houses and a parent who smoked. Bronchitis falls into two types: acute, that's where a viral infection is the cause or the bronchial tract has become irritated; and chronic, which results from prolonged exposure to irritants. As I have found out myself, there are ways to prevent it. So let's look at them first.

PREVENTION: Okay, what I said about damp houses and smoking parents is true to a certain extent. Children are more likely to develop bronchitis if their parents smoke so if this is you, then try not to do so in their presence, or in rooms they are likely to be in. Also, going further back to when your child was born, there are studies that show that breast-fed babies are less likely to develop respiratory infections during childhood. In some instances, acute bronchitis develops from a cold or flu. If you have those then don't neglect them. Chronic bronchitis is often associated with an allergy, as it were, to certain chemicals, or to smoke – sometimes even from passive smoking. So if you know what causes it try to avoid it, or you're going to go on damaging your system. A diet high in antioxidants can help. Eating lots of fish, fruit and vegetables in particular can help with chronic bronchitis, as can taking vitamin C supplements, while taking too much sugar or dairy products can make it worse.

HOREHOUND: This herb is good for coughs. Try two teaspoons in a cup of boiling water with a dash of lemon juice. Allow to steep for 15 minutes, then drink.

MAGNESIUM: Make sure you have plenty of this your diet, as the more there is the less likelihood there is of you wheezing through another attack! An excellent source is nuts. (See Magnesium, page 198.)

IVY: Useful for treating a dose of bronchitis. (See Ivy, page 190.)

MARSH MALLOW: This was used for centuries to treat bronchitis and is quite easy to come by. Although you can take tablets, sometimes a cup of tea is best to help soothe the throat. (See Marsh mallow, page 200.)

LOBELIA: This herb contains many anti-inflammatory properties making it useful for treating this condition. Ask at your health shop for preparations containing it.

EUCALYPTUS: Inhaling eucalyptus oil can help clear the blocked passages. Simply pour some in boiling water, put a towel over your head and inhale. Or burn some in the sick room. (See Eucalyptus, page 164.)

GARLIC: Either take garlic with your food or buy the capsules. Nowadays they're even odourless in some instances. (See Garlic, page 174.)

LICORICE: Licorice is an anti-inflammatory, just what you need for this condition. (See Licorice, page 195.)

THYME: I would recommend a cup of thyme tea to help soothe your sore throat. Thyme was used for centuries in the treatment of bronchitis and various studies show it's as effective as other drugs. (See Thyme, page 236.)

ELDERBERRY: This one's for flu but as many of the symptoms are similar, I wouldn't hesitate to use it. (See Elderberry, page 163.)

ECHINACEA: This is excellent for boosting the immune system, thus helping you over a dose of bronchitis. It's also to be recommended for helping to stop you having another attack if taken regularly. (See Echinacea, page 161.)

A WORD OF CAUTION: Please refer to the individual supplements and take according to the instructions. Also, if your condition is not clearing or seems to be getting worse, seek medical advice.

INTERESTING FACT: The Chinese recommend honeysuckle tea for bronchitis. I think that sounds so much better than the goose grease, mustard and brown paper poultices that were stuck on the chest with candle wax by people in Britain centuries ago!

Bruises

Bruises are caused by blood leaking under the skin, usually after an injury. But sometimes larger ones can be painful and tender to the touch, as well as being unsightly. There's nothing worse than sporting the traditional 'keeker' or 'shiner' (i.e. a black eye) just when you want to look your best.

PREVENTION: Well really, that's very difficult. Well nigh impossible in fact. I will say, however, that some people bruise more easily than others. For those with that problem, eating pineapple regularly is said to help. That's because it contains substances that strengthen the capillaries, thus preventing too many leakages. If someone has hurt themselves a good trick is to place an ice-pack on the area in question even before it has a chance to bruise significantly. Then you can treat it with one of the following.

POTATO: Never mind the steak! I've heard it said that popping a raw potato on a black eye is just as effective, as well as being a whole lot cheaper.

WITCH HAZEL: This is one of those traditional skin remedies that is excellent for many things, including bruises! In addition to helping them heal quickly, it soothes the tender painful feeling. (See Witch hazel, page 252.)

COMFREY: This is also an old remedy for bruises. One that goes back hundreds of years. Nowadays you don't have to boil the plant, you can just look in your health shop for a cream containing it and save yourself a lot of trouble.

LAVENDER: Lavender is a good healing herb. You can make a tea by pouring boiling water over some crushed lavender. It's very effective if you add a little crushed parsley. Then just gently dab it on. Or you can try dabbing a little lavender oil onto the area. (See Lavender, page 192.)

ROSEMARY: If you try adding a little rosemary oil to a vegetable oil base and massaging it into the bruise, it should help.

OATMEAL: Poultices of oatmeal were a traditional method of treating bruises. Make a mash with hot water and apply.

A WORD OF CAUTION: Please don't take any of the above remedies. All are intended for external use only. Serious unexplained bruising can sometimes be the sign of other conditions and should be checked by your doctor.

INTERESTING FACT: Traditionally, St John's Wort was regarded as the best cure for bruises, simply because when it is roughly handled, this plant oozes red oil, much as the skin does when it bruises!

Bunions

A large bump at the foot of the big toe, a bunion is sometimes caused by a hereditary weakness called Hallux Valgus, but more commonly by ill-fitting shoes, so prevention being better than cure, always make sure your shoes fit and that they do not rub the side of the feet.

Once there, bunions are for keeps, unless surgically removed and, however they are caused, can become painful, especially if a sufferer is on their feet too long.

Turmeric, camomile and pineapple are all good for easing the 'nip' all sufferers complain of at one time or another and are very easy to find and take.

TURMERIC: Turmeric has a rather hot, burning sensation, so unless you want your mouth to feel as if you've eaten six curries in a row, this hot herb should be taken in capsule form daily.

PINEAPPLE: Fresh pineapple seasoned with ginger is delicious and, eaten regularly, is a good way of keeping inflammation down.

CAMOMILE: Camomile, too, has the same soothing properties and can be drunk as a tea. You can even be really disgusting and squeeze the bag on the bunion when you've done! (See Camomile, page 145)

Burns

Burns come in all degrees and obviously if you have been severely burned then the place for you is a hospital. What I'm looking at here are 'minor' burns, the kind caused by touching a hot oven, or pot. Burns are of course very painful, whether 'minor' or not and quite hard to treat in terms of stopping the skin breaking and then going septic. Small burns can be held under the cold tap. This helps moisturise the skin and calm things down. You can then place a dry piece of lint over it to keep it covered. Other things you can use are:

ALOE VERA: The gel is good for skin whether sunburnt or not and I have used it to treat household burns when there is nothing else at hand. Not only did it help the burn heal, it also prevented the skin blistering and peeling. (See Aloe Vera, page 121.)

CUCUMBER: You can try slicing a cucumber and placing it on the affected area. Cucumbers are very good for skin care. In particular they keep the skin moist, always a problem when it has been damaged.

CALENDULA: A cream containing calendula or marigold can be applied to a burn. Just dab it on with a little cotton wool. If the skin does break it will act as a good antiseptic. (See Calendula, page 144.)

CAMOMILE: You can try dabbing a little camomile tea on the burn in much the same way as Calendula. Just make sure it has cooled of course, otherwise that won't just be a burn but a scald. (See Camomile, page 145.)

A WORD OF CAUTION: Please refer to the individual remedy for any cautions.

INTERESTING FACT: Pastes made of baking soda spread on gauze and applied to a burn were a favourite Victorian way of dealing with burns. I've actually tried this and guess what? Not only did the burn heal rapidly but the skin didn't break at all.

Candida

We all have a certain amount of yeast on the moist parts of our bodies, which generally does no harm. Only there are times when we have more than usual and it causes an infection. Sometimes certain medicines cause the yeast to get out of hand, or it could be other allergies. I had it when I was pregnant, probably because of the hormonal changes to the body. I also know of women who have suffered constantly since going through the menopause. Women in the main tend to suffer but if you have it the chances are your partner does too. It's just that men often don't have any symptoms. So if you're a woman, looking at this page and thinking 'I have candida,' then unless your partner is treated too, you're going to be re-infected. The main symptom of candida is an unbearable vaginal itch, accompanied by a hot burning sensation, odour and discharge. Yeast infections can also develop in the mouth and on the skin, anywhere that tends to be moist. If you suspect you have one you should see a doctor. That's the first step. The chances are that they will prescribe something for you. There are, however, certain herbal remedies you could try and also certain things you can look at if you tend to be a regular sufferer or, even worse, can't get an infection to go away as often happens.

PREVENTION: You sometimes can't stop something like this from striking, but you can be aware that it seems to be changes to the body's natural balance that trigger it. Therefore it would make sense to include certain basic yeast inhibitors in your diet. I didn't know about them when I was a sufferer. Now I do and you can bet they're in mine!

CRANBERRY: Cranberries are good for a variety of things. They possess a compound that treats candida. (See Cranberry, page 155.)

GARLIC: Since garlic stops fungi growing, it can be effective here. What's more, you don't have to go eating up leaves or chopping up cloves if you don't want to. You can get garlic tablets from your supermarket or health shop and take according to instructions. Generally, including garlic in your food is good for you. I do it all the time, be it rice, pasta, pizza, whatever. There's no vampires to be seen round my kitchen, I can tell you! (See Garlic, page 174.)

SAGE: Mint plants can stop mould growing and sage is a member of that family. I would certainly recommend a cup of sage tea or even a sage bath to help this condition. (See Sage, page 227.)

MINT (SPEARMINT): Given mint's ability to stop cheese going mouldy, I even think it would be worth a try here. At least I don't think it would do any harm to try a mint tea or running the bath water through some leaves.

ECHINACEA: This can be very useful here. Many studies show that it reduces yeast infections. (See Echinacea, page 161.)

IVY: A pinch of dried herb in hot water can help, or it might be more appropriate to ask at your health shop for a tincture containing it. (See Ivy, page 190.)

TEA TREE OIL: While tea tree oil must never be taken orally, it can help fight candida. (See Tea tree oil, page 233.)

A WORD OF CAUTION: Please refer to the individual instructions for each remedy above and follow these. Obviously, if you have a problem using a particular herb then stop using it. Remember, too, that if you suspect you have candida, please see a doctor first. The vagina is a very sensitive area and I don't want you getting into a terrible mess because you've tried to treat something that may not be candida at all. If you're going to try some of the diet suggestions, then be patient too. I know this is difficult with this condition, but for things to build up in the system takes time. However, if you're a long-term sufferer and in despair, the diet remedies are worth looking at.

INTERESTING FACT: Sometimes rubbing on yoghurt is recommended. After all it's bound to be full of things that stop it going mouldy!

Conjunctivitis

Conjunctivitis – pinkeye or redeye – is an inflammation of the membranes that line the eye, which can sometimes cause it to become so swollen and painful that the sufferer can't see out of it. We all know what it's like when we get a bit of grit in our eye.

That's bad enough. However, in really severe cases of conjunctivitis, a sufferer's face can swell, the eye won't stop running and, of course, because it's itchy, you want to scratch and that makes it worse. While antibiotics can help in some instances, they don't work right away and the infection often returns. So here are some tips.

PREVENTION: If you have a sufferer in your family, indeed if you suffer yourself, make sure you don't share face cloths or towels. When you wash your face, dab the affected side dry with a different towel because, yes, the infection can be spread and this is the most common way of doing so. In some cases the sufferer is allergic to a substance – it could be chlorine in the swimming pool. So try to identify what that substance might be and stay away from it. If you have a bit of grit in your eye, remove it carefully and gently with a small piece of wet cotton wool. Don't poke or rub. That just makes it go in further and irritates the eye.

DIET: In some instances, people who are chronic sufferers have a vitamin A deficiency, although it's not clear if upping your intake will help. I would say it's still worth a try. Anything is if this is a problem that won't go away. (See Vitamin A, page 240.)

EYEBRIGHT: I think you can tell from the name that this might just be for the eyes? In olden times, people used to name herbs after the things they could help. So I think we can take it as read that this will help you. Although I must add at this stage that there are no scientific studies on the use of this herb. If you want to try it, ask for a tincture at your health shop and apply according to instructions. In case you can't see too well at the time, that will mean putting some drops in water and carefully dabbing it on. When you apply, be sure you dispose of the cloth and use a fresh one if your other eye is infected.

GOLDENSEAL: This one is good for reducing inflammation, especially of the mucous membranes. Ask at your health shop for an ointment containing it, although you might also find the tablets helpful.

CAMOMILE: Camomile has traditionally been used for eye ailments. Make a cup of tea with camomile tea bags, allow too cool and carefully apply to the eye. You can even try just applying the bags and drinking the tea. Repeat as often as necessary. (See Camomile, page 145.)

COMFREY: Applied externally, comfrey is a useful herb for this condition. (See Comfrey, page 154.)

A WORD OF CAUTION: Please remember these are your eyes we're talking about here. At the risk of sounding like a Disney World ride guide, approach remedies with care, and according to the instructions. If your condition starts to improve, then you can try using more of the remedy you choose, if it doesn't, or seems to flare, discontinue use immediately.

INTERESTING FACT: Conjunctivitis is one of those ailments for which very little research has been done.

Constipation

Well, here's another 'bane', so to speak. And, sadly, this is a condition that is mainly confined to us folk here in the West because of diet and lifestyle. If people ate properly, this condition would almost vanish overnight. Having said that, sometimes constipation is the sign of a much more serious condition. So if having had very little history of it before, you suddenly find yourself suffering badly from it for no apparent reason you can think of (e.g. diet, illness or medication), then you should see a doctor. When treating general constipation it's important to look at different things and take them into account. That's because there are different types. Most importantly, too, you should look at your diet. A lot of money is spent on laxatives, which often just solve the problem for a day or so. Then, because the system has overexerted itself, you become constipated again and 'addictions' set in. In the long run that doesn't help – sorry, no pun intended!

PREVENTION: Most cases of constipation are caused by insufficient fibre in the diet. If you do nothing but eat lots of meat, fatty substances and dairy foods, and sit about all day, then there's not much doubt that you are going to be constipated. Even if you don't sit about all day, you are going to be constipated. You are going to be constipated because what you should be doing is eating more fruit (in particular, grapes, apples, pineapples), vegetables, cereals, brown wholemeal bread and drinking lots of water and orange juice. Okay, so you don't have to eat and drink your way through everything I've suggested, becoming a health freak overnight! But the first thing to look at is your diet. Not only is constipation a Western disease, so is diverticulitis, which is largely caused by years of eating insufficient fibre diets and lots of processed foods. The latter is another thing we're very into, often because our lives are so busy. It's so much easier, isn't it, to open a packet. And there's nothing wrong with doing that, provided that's being balanced with fresh food. Even just making a small change, such as starting the day on a glass of fresh orange and a bowl of cereal, can help. Diet is very important, too, in instances where illness is involved and you're lying in bed, unable to get up and move about. Often in these instances constipation results, so make sure you take plenty of vegetable soups.

Children often have quite appalling diets. A succession of crisps, biscuits and other things make their way into their little tums! It's amazing in some instances their systems work at all. And as any long-suffering mum will know, it's so hard to get them to eat the right things. One of mine lived for six years entirely on digestive biscuits. At least they were wholemeal! But I used to dread when she went to school and opened her lunchbox, in case the teachers thought I was starving her. How she ever lived at all is beyond me. But joking apart – and I'm not – try to encourage children to eat fruit and vegetables from an early age. I did and it got me nowhere. But not to worry. There's always good children's cereals and, when they're old enough not to choke on them, peanuts and beans, even baked ones. If you have a liquidiser you can always make tempting things like your own ice-cream, by simmering your choice of fresh fruit in a little sugar, whisking, chilling, then whisking again with double cream and freezing. Okay, so that's a brief look at some dietary tips, but if you're really stuck and you want some natural advice on what to do now I've outlined some remedies below.

PRUNE JUICE: Absolutely revolting, I have to say, but a very good laxative, apparently, if you are really stuck! If you have a liquidiser you can mash your own.

BRAN: Regular daily intake keeps the system in good working order and is very easy to come by either in bread or as a cereal. (See Bran, page 137.)

FRESH ORANGE JUICE: This is good for getting a sluggish system to work naturally.

RHUBARB: This is a natural laxative and rather powerful too. Either eat it raw or stew it with a little sugar and water.

DANDELION: Dandelion is useful for many things and constipation is one of them. But you need the root extract. Ask at your health shop. (See Dandelion, page 159.)

LICORICE: Chew a licorice stick. The kind bought from a health shop. (See Licorice, page 195.)

ALOE VERA: This is very good for chronic constipation and detoxing the system generally. You would need to buy the juice from a health shop, however, and it is rather pricey. (See Aloe Vera, page 121.)

PSYLLIUM: Taking three to ten tablespoons a day of psyllium seeds can get the bowels moving, but you have to take a lot of water too, in case the digestive system gets damaged. It's also not a suitable remedy if you have asthma.

A WORD OF CAUTION: Please check the individual remedy for any cautions. If your constipation persists, see a doctor. As I said before, if you are suffering a prolonged bout and this is unusual for you, see a doctor in case you have an obstruction. Look to improving your diet in other instances. Prolonged use of laxatives can become addictive and harm the system. Continual constipation caused by poor diet often results in other conditions.

INTERESTING FACT: In countries where the diet is full of berry fruit, nuts and pulses, constipation is unknown. But then some of them have rather high rates of diarrhoea.

Corns

Corns can be the bane of your life, or rather your feet. They are thickened areas of skin on the toes, generally of a conical shape. The 'eye' or tip points in, causing pain.

PREVENTION: Prevention is always better than cure. As with many foot problems, the best thing is to stop them forming in the first place and the best way to do this is to wear properly fitting shoes. Shoes that are too small and bunch the toes will generally result in corns as well as other painful conditions (see Bunions, page 130). Take care of your feet. Think of all the time you are on them. If you stand a lot, wear a flattish shoe. Personally I adore a heel, but some of the towering heights presently being manufactured in the name of fashion look to me as if they could cause all kinds of problems. And not just for the feet. So be sensible.

FIG: The pulp of a fresh fig can help remove a corn. (See Figs, page 170.)

WINTERGREEN: Ask at your health shop for wintergreen ointment or oil and try applying it to the corn. Remember this means the corn only, not the surrounding skin. It should help relieve the pain and dissolve the hardened skin. You can then rub away what's left with a pumice stone.

HOT WATER: You can always try putting your foot in hot soapy water then gently scraping the hard skin away with a pair of scissors, then a pumice stone. But you might have to do this several times, over a period of time to remove the corn and it depends how patient you are. Dry, then cover with a plaster.

A WORD OF WARNING: Do not feel tempted to take the wintergreen oil internally just because it smells nice. These kinds of oil are intended for external use only. Remember, if you're scraping your foot, do so with clean materials and do not prod or poke, in case you set up some kind of infection.

INTERESTING FACT: Oscar Wilde must have known a thing or two about corns and sensitivity. In his deliciously wicked way, he defined a 'sensitive' person as someone 'who, because he has corns himself, always treads on other people's toes'.

Cough

Most of us can't get through the winter without developing a cold, and one of the most annoying symptoms of that is a cough, particularly one that won't clear. Flu can also leave a lingering 'hacker' that goes on for weeks and, if you're bronchial, sometimes just being in a change of temperature can trigger one off. Any cough that goes on too long, or produces blood-stained mucus, requires a trip to the doctor's. If you're worried, always consult a medical professional. Some herbs do have a history of treating a cough and you might find them helpful if you've caught a cold.

ELDERBERRY: Elderberry is very useful for treating a cough and helping with colds in general. You can look for a cough medicine containing it, or buy a tincture from your health shop and keep it handy, using it as directed. A nice hot drink containing a few drops and some lemon, water and honey taken at bedtime should help soothe your throat and let you get to sleep.

EUCALYPTUS: This is especially helpful for loosening up mucus. However, remember to inhale only. (See Eucalyptus, page 164.)

MARSH MALLOW: No, it's not just a sweet! The root is very good for treating irritation associated with a dry tickly cough. Ask at your health shop for the dried herb, then you can make a tea. It's not a case of eating lots of it and hoping for the best!

LICORICE: Licorice too isn't just a sweet. Traditionally, it was used to treat coughs and asthma. But before you go rushing to the sweet shop, thinking 'I'm going to enjoy this' – stop! What you need are the extracts from the root. Again, you will have to visit your health store to see what they have on offer, or check the contents on some of the herbal cough medicines. If licorice is included, it's a good bet. (See Licorice, page 195.)

NETTLE: So you think all the stinging bits would be the worst thing to take for an irritated throat? Think again. Nettle was traditionally used to cure coughs and colds. Once they are boiled, the leaves lose their sting. That's providing you don't get stung first, however! Then there's the problem of what may have been sprayed on them! Ask at your health shop for extracts. (See Nettle, page 207.)

THYME: Due to its low toxicity this is a favourite for treating children's coughs. Put a teaspoon in a cup of boiling water for ten minutes. Strain, then drink. You can also try inhaling the vapours. Put a spoonful in a basin, cover your head with a towel and inhale.

A WORD OF CAUTION: Licorice can cause headaches, when taken to excess. If your cough has persisted for weeks, consult your doctor.

INTERESTING FACT: Other traditional cough remedies include lobelia and coltsfoot.

Cramp

At some time or other, unless we're incredibly lucky, the chances are we're going to suffer from cramp and a very alarming experience it can be too. Agony in fact. The funny thing being that, on the whole, it's not a serious condition (i.e. not one that's likely to kill you, unless your toes happen to cramp when you're crossing the road and then you're stuck there). Yes, it's happened to me and very silly I looked too. With cramp, the muscles knot and tend to stay knotted for a time, so any movement is painful. Usually it is just the body's way of responding to being over-exerted in some way, hence the amount of athletes who suffer.

However, there are some good herbal remedies. Some I swear by myself and others I have recommended to clients.

PREVENTION: Some night-time leg cramps are caused by poor circulation and simply by being cold. Make sure you're warm at night, so you won't wake up writhing about the bed in agony. Or wear socks. Who cares if it's not glamorous! So long as it helps stop cramps, that's what counts! Stomach cramps, on the other hand, are often caused by eating in an unnatural position, bolting food or being in a state of tension. If this is you, then perhaps you're needing to look at your eating habits. Athletes often experience cramp because they sweat heavily, leading to a salt deficiency. This can be helped by drinking plenty of fluids before competing or taking salt tablets. Persistent cramp may be the sign of a vitamin or mineral deficiency, one that may be caused by poor diet. (See the sections on Vitamins, Magnesium and Calcium to see if you are getting enough from your food.) For menstrual cramps, please refer to that section.

MYRRH: Rubbing a few drop of essential myrrh oil into the muscle or putting some on a hot, damp cloth, then applying to the limb, should help ease the ache.

GARLIC: Garlic is good for the circulation, so taking garlic capsules daily may help this problem if you tend to suffer a lot. (See Garlic, page 174.)

NETTLE: Because nettle contains a high proportion of minerals, it is another one that could help if taken regularly. I would suggest taking it here as a tea. Boil a handful of leaves in 1 litre of water. Leave to stand for ten minutes, strain then drink one cup twice a day. (See Nettle, page 207.)

BLACK COHOSH: This is also good for the relief of cramps and one I personally recommend. (See Black cohosh, page 135.)

FEVERFEW: Taking feverfew capsules could help stop you suffering cramps. Feverfew's many compounds are good for a variety of ailments of this kind. (See Feverfew, page 169.)

A WORD OF CAUTION: Please refer to the particular herb you intend to use to see which is suitable, as some are more use than others and some cannot be used if you are pregnant or breastfeeding.

INTERESTING FACT: Traditionally, magnets were strapped to the affected joint to relieve the pain. This isn't one I would recommend!

Dandruff

Well, this can be the plague of many a scalp! Sometimes you aren't even the one who notices it. It's the person behind you in the bus queue. Or, if you don't take the bus, the cinema. Wherever. It's the person behind you full stop. Dandruff is when the scalp flakes. Just when we were trying to look drop-dead gorgeous too! But the only thing dropping is the dead skin. Sometimes the scalp is itchy. When something is itchy the first rule is to scratch. Then, in some instances, we've a fine mess on our hands! What can we do? Well, there are lots of anti-dandruff shampoos on the market, but if you're reading this, the chances are you want to know about herbal remedies. The good news is that there are a great many herbal shampoos now available, as there are with other body products. So you can find one that is suitable, or add the recommended herbs to your own personal favourite.

TEA TREE OIL: The disinfectant substances in tea tree penetrate the scalp far deeper than any other. What's more, it's now available as a shampoo. If the scalp is broken, however, I will warn you that it will sting. So be prepared to go through the ceiling! If not, this is a good one for treating dandruff and preventing its return. (See Tea tree oil, page 233.)

COMFREY: Either look for a shampoo containing it or add a few drops of tincture to your normal shampoo. Comfrey has anti-dandruff properties. (See Comfrey, page 154.)

LICORICE: The dried herb contains properties that stop the scalp secreting so much oil, then flaking. Ask at your health shop for a tincture to add to your existing shampoo, or for a packet of the dried herb. Steeped in vinegar it can be used as a rinse. (See Licorice, page 196.)

OLIVE OIL: You can try removing dry dandruff with olive oil. Heat the oil by standing it in a bowl of hot water, then apply with a pad of cotton wool to the scalp and roots of the hair. Wrap the head in a towel and leave on for three hours. This sounds a lot but it's a great excuse to watch your favourite video. Shampoo off thoroughly.

A WORD OF CAUTION: Do not try to take tea tree oil or comfrey. These are intended for external use only. Remember, we should treat all herbal medicines with respect and not just assume they aren't powerful. They are. That's why they work!

INTERESTING FACT: Vinegar and apple cider were used traditionally to treat dandruff. Warm both, apply to the scalp, then shampoo.

Depression

The other day someone said to me, 'You're so good at your job. You have everything under control.' But I'm not. I'm hopeless. I know they're just saying that. I used to like going out, but now I can't be bothered. It's such an effort getting ready and there's no point. I never look good anyhow. That dress I bought the other day shows all my fat and I don't know what to say to people. I don't have an interesting life and I know they're really thinking, 'Huh, she's hopeless. She can't do anything.' And I can't. That's the truth. I'm useless. There are times I even want to end it. I don't see the point continuing. I want to walk into the river and feel the water going over my head … Okay, got your attention have I? Well that's good because I'm not actually talking about myself. I'm talking about depression. Something that at its best might mean you not being able to make the meal tonight and at worst can lead you to that river and make you walk in. You feel so worthless. I don't know if I can help, but I would like to try. Bear in mind there are many causes of depression. Let's take a look at them.

UNDERSTANDING DEPRESSION: When you're depressed it's very hard to see how you got there or how to get out. In some instances, it is just a mood swing, a one-off. But that's very few instances, I have to say. Some depression can actually be caused, not by physical events such as the death of a close one, as you might suspect, but by thyroid malfunction. If your thyroid is set on low, then it can result in depression. What it needs is correcting. Depression caused by stressful events, such as loss or death, is often best treated by counselling, by talking things out of your system, by seeking new interests and friends. Setting yourself realistic daily targets in terms of things to achieve is a good idea. Exercise has been shown to be helpful because it helps the body release substances that can relieve depression. In some instances, depression is caused by an allergy to certain foodstuffs. Cutting down on the sugar and caffeine can be helpful. Life's little pleasures, eh! Alcohol, which is something many depressed people turn to, can often make things worse.

Sometimes depression is actually a sign of something else, such as a hormonal imbalance. When you think of the amount of menopausal women who get depressed, it's possible that what they are suffering is linked to this. Similarly oral contraceptives have been shown to cause deficiencies of certain vitamins that are necessary for normal functioning. Vitamin B6 is one of those. Dietary deficiencies in vitamin B12, folic acid, and Omega-3 fatty acids, can all lead to disturbing mood swings. A great many people with depression have actually been found to have at least one of these deficiencies. So it might do you good to read the sections on these and check out whether you think you are deficient. Sometimes what you've thought of as a 'mental' problem is actually much more physical.

ST JOHN'S WORT: This has been shown to help symptoms of worthlessness and anxiety so many times, it's almost the herbal Prozac! It's one I often recommend, in certain conditions of course, and to find out what they are, see the section on Dr Bach's Flower Remedies on pages 102–3 and page 130.

ROSEMARY: The oil is a favourite with aromatherapists for treating a number of things, one of which happens to be depression. That's because it stimulates the central nervous system. You could try burning it regularly, or massaging it into your skin. (See Rosemary, page 226.)

GINGKO BILOBA: Here's another that's also good for a number of ailments. Try taking 80 ml a day and see if that improves your state of mind. (See Gingko biloba, page 177.)

GINGER: You could try taking a capsule a day if you are depressed or adding the herb to your food.

A WORD OF CAUTION: Depression is a hard thing to fight. Remember we all experience feelings of uselessness at some stage in our lives. You are never alone in that regard. Hopefully you will find that some of the things suggested will help. If they don't and you feel yourself sliding all the way to the brink, see a doctor.

INTERESTING FACT: A wort, as in St John's Wort, is actually a plant, in case you were wondering.

Diarrhoea

Well, everyone knows what this is – gippy tummy, Delhi belly, holiday ruination, whatever it's called – so I'm not going to go into the gory details. Continual diarrhoea is sometimes the sign of a digestive problem that needs checked out by a doctor, as does infant diarrhoea. Children become dehydrated very quickly. Indeed we all do, so it's very important, if you have diarrhoea, to drink lots of fluids. It's important, too, in some instances, to take rehydration drinks because, in severe cases, vital minerals are also being lost from the system. Fortunately, no matter how unpleasant, most cases of diarrhoea tend to clear up within 48 hours and there are things you can take that help settle the system. Diarrhoea is the body's way of getting rid of bacteria – although it's difficult to take comfort from this at the time!

PREVENTION: Diarrhoea tends to strike holidaymakers. It's like a little 'welcome to the country!'. Watch what you eat and drink if you're abroad. However, it's a fact that even drinking bottled water can give you the runs, simply because the system isn't accustomed to that kind of water, amount of minerals, etc. So often it's simply 'the change' of everything that's doing it. Some foods do have a laxative effect too. If you eat a plate of prunes or figs, for example, there's no point complaining! Rich fatty foods do much the same. When preparing food always make sure that your hands, surfaces and utensils are clean. Cook according to instructions. Store food – uncooked, cooked, fresh or frozen – properly, making sure you throw out things that are past their sell-by date. If you leave a pot of cooked meat out on the cooker, with no lid on and come back to it the next day, thinking 'I'll just have this now,' have it you will – diarrhoea, I mean. I wouldn't like to tell you about all the nasties that will have settled on the meat in the meantime! While a certain amount of dirt can be good for us, keep your standards high for bathrooms and kitchens! Also, some cases of diarrhoea are caused by stress – bolting food, not eating properly and chucking anything down our throats. So, if this sounds like you, then you know what to do!

APPLE: Apples are good for both constipation and diarrhoea and traditionally have been used for both too.

BLACKBERRY: A cup or two of blackberry tea can help soothe an upset stomach, as well as keeping your fluid intake level up. (See Blackberry, page 136.)

CAMOMILE: This herb is a gentle relaxant. So if you've got your system in a state through stress or anxiety, then I'd recommend you sit down and drink a cup. (See Camomile, page 145.)

BILBERRY: Dried bilberry is very good for relieving diarrhoea. That's because it's full of pectin. (See Bilberry, page 134.)

CARROT: A plate of carrots can soothe the digestive system as well as provide it with important nutrients.

THYME: Thyme can settle a churning stomach and kill bacteria. Pour a cup of boiling water over a teaspoon of the herb, steep, strain and drink. (See Thyme, page 236.)

A WORD OF CAUTION: Please refer to the individual remedy. Persistent diarrhoea sufferers or people experiencing sudden changes in their bowel habits should see their doctor as this could be the sign of a stomach disorder or disease.

INTERESTING FACT: Laudanum was the great Victorian cure for diarrhoea.

Dry mouth

Not only is a dry mouth unpleasant, it can be bad for you. We all need the saliva to flow. It helps control germs in the mouth, preventing tooth decay and gum disease. So if you're a sufferer, don't ignore it. A lot of people with dry mouth are people who use their voices in their occupations. After a day with clients, I'm a sufferer myself, I can tell you. I've a large tank of water in the office to prove it! If you're in this category, even keeping a glass of water handy and sipping it regularly can help prevent the saliva from drying. Water is much better than a manufactured drink, which might contain sugar, as that dries the mouth further. Smoking, too, doesn't help. If you're speaking constantly and the first thing you do when you finish is reach for a cigarette, then you're aggravating not only your mouth but your throat, making you more prone to conditions that affect it. Sometimes, too, certain medicines cause a dry mouth. It's one of the side effects unfortunately. Also, if we're in a stressful situation, or feeling nervous for whatever reason, the glands seem to dry up of their own accord. Again, try and have water to hand, or a damp handkerchief to wet the lips.

ECHINACEA: Even a drop of this herb in a cup of tea or juice, can help bring relief to sufferers. Echinacea contains a compound that produces saliva. (See Echinacea, page 161.)

EVENING PRIMROSE OIL: This is readily obtainable from supermarkets and health shops in capsule form and is also good for relieving a dry mouth. (See Evening primrose oil, page 165.)

RED PEPPER (CAYENNE POWDER): Some people swear by red pepper for stimulating the salivary glands in the mouth. Onion probably has the same effect. If you eat lots of both regularly you might find the problem is eased.

A WORD OF WARNING: If you are constantly thirsty in addition to having a dry mouth, please consult your doctor, as this can be a sign of other things that may or may not be serious.

INTERESTING FACT: The Indians of South America have a special plant to cure dry mouth called jaborandi, which means 'that which causes slobbering'. If you think of the word 'jabber' it probably means much the same. Let's face it, it's far easier to do when your mouth isn't dry!

Eczema

The main symptom of eczema is an itchy, red rash. But then so is the symptom of lots of other skin conditions. It's important you don't make things worse by using the wrong ointment or treatment, so the first thing you should do is have it properly diagnosed by a doctor. That way you know what you're dealing with. Then you'll know how to start treating it. Skin problems are difficult, which I think you'll know if you've got one. Just when you think it's going away, it flares. Sometimes there's a reason for that, so let's take a look.

PREVENTION: In many instances, eczema is triggered by an allergy – food allergies in particular. It's therefore important that you find out what causes it to flare and cut it from your diet. One study shows that when certain sufferers cut out coffee, their symptoms improved. Maybe in your case it's worth giving this a try. Other research suggests that certain additions to the diet can help. Vitamin E is widely touted as being beneficial to skin complaints, as is vitamin B complex. So is the trace mineral zinc. And I would refer you to the appropriate sections on these. Eating plenty of fish is good, as are pineapples, oranges and carrots. It has also been noted that many people with eczema can't process their fatty acids properly, resulting in a deficiency, in which case taking evening primrose oil is thought to be helpful. Other things include:

ALOE VERA: Not just for sunburn, Aloe Vera is very effective for treating most skin problems. Just apply the gel to the affected area twice a day. (See Aloe Vera, page 121.)

CALENDULA: Calendula gets the white blood cells going so that they speed healing generally. Look for a cream or ointment containing it. (See Calendula, page 144.)

CARROT: In addition to being good to eat, carrots are excellent for the skin if you make them into a mash and apply.

PANSY: Very useful for treating many skin conditions, including this one. Make a tea with the petals and leaves by steeping them in boiling water, steep, then strain and when cool apply to the affected area.

COMFREY: Creams containing comfrey are useful for treating eczema. If you can't get one but can get a tincture instead, then you could put a few drops in water and apply. (See Comfrey, page 154.)

A WORD OF CAUTION: Please refer to the individual remedy for any cautions, and never take anything that is meant for external use.

INTERESTING FACTS: Those Egyptian pharaohs knew their stuff. They liked to bathe in Aloe Vera to keep their skin looking good. Given the cost of doing that nowadays you'd need a pharaoh's fortune. Cleopatra used sour milk.

Fainting

Fainting is a temporary loss of consciousness caused by a decreased blood flow to the brain. Victorian women were especially good at it, I reckon because their corsets were too tight, rather than that the men were so handsome! But if it happens to you, or someone collapses in front of you, it's rather worrying and good to know what to do.

PREVENTION: Hunger, exhaustion, severe emotional upset and being in a hot stuffy environment can do it. First you feel dizzy, then you lose consciousness. Eat regularly. If you feel hungry and light headed, do something about it immediately. Make sure the room you are in is well aired and you don't feel hot. If you feel faint or are with someone who does, sit with the head lowered between the knees, or lie with the legs elevated, to get more blood to the brain. Loosen tight clothing. If the person is hot and you can get a cool cloth for the head, or wrists, then do so.

COFFEE: A cup of coffee is good for someone who has fainted or feels faint. It's not just an old wives' tale. The caffeine helps stimulate the body generally.

ROSEMARY: If someone faints, place a drop of rosemary oil, or even a piece of crushed herb, under their nose. Of course, we don't all go about carrying such things, as the Victorians did, but you could have a small sachet in your pocket, say of rosemary and dried lavender, to use if you or anyone else felt faint. (See Rosemary, page 226.)

LAVENDER: (See Lavender, page 192.)

EUCALYPTUS: Eucalyptus oil has much the same qualities as rosemary. A drop or two on a cloth can soon revive a person who has fainted and a cup of eucalyptus tea is very good for getting them back on their feet. (See Eucalyptus, page 164.)

A WORD OF CAUTION: Never give anyone eucalyptus, rosemary or lavender oil to swallow. It can be very harmful. We can all faint from the above causes, but if this is happening to you regularly then please see a doctor. Some of the things that cause fainting are serious.

INTERESTING FACT: Women did faint more often in the Victorian days than any other time. It was termed 'swooning'.

Flatulence

Well, this is an embarrassing one. Of course a certain amount is normal, you just can't stop the food you eat producing gas. But sometimes, let's be honest, you can eat something that murders your insides, causing severe pain and bloating. Then there are times when you get trapped wind and it causes niggling shooting pains throughout your stomach and often up into your ribcage as well. At worst you actually think something is seriously wrong. So what can you do about this little problem?

PREVENTION: Well, it's true that certain foodstuffs are very gassy. Beans in particular, if you remember the scene in *Blazing Saddles*. Green vegetables and starchy foods are other offenders. Often these foodstuffs are so good in other ways, though, it's a shame to cut them out. Cutting down might be more helpful. Also, if you find a certain foodstuff doesn't agree with you, then stop eating it. A good thing to try by way of lessening flatulence is to make sure you chew your food thoroughly. That way you should cut down on bloating, indigestion and the nasty little problem I'm talking about here.

BLESSED THISTLE: Try keeping some tablets handy as you would other stomach remedies. Then if you are troubled, you can try taking one.

RED PEPPER (CAYENNE POWDER): This is excellent for many ailments and, although hot and spicy, actually isn't a culprit in the wind stakes. Try sprinkling it on your cooking, or buy cayenne capsules and keep them handy for when you suffer. (See Red pepper, page 220.)

PARSLEY: This is another help, which benefits digestion. Some people deliberately keep a piece till last, when they see it on a salad. You should try doing the same. Or go one better and have a plant in your garden. Then you'll always have some available for this problem. (See Parsley, page 213.)

VALERIAN: Valerian has many calming qualities and can be used for an upset stomach or wind. Just put five drops in a little water and drink. You should certainly start to feel better fairly quickly. (See Valerian, page 239.)

A WORD OF CAUTION: Please refer to the appropriate remedy for any cautions.

INTERESTING FACT: The Victorians took a teaspoon of cinnamon to expel their gas. You're quite welcome to try but please note the emphasis is on expel.

Flu

If you're unlucky enough to get it, flu is an absolute misery. That's if you're relatively healthy. For the young, the old, those with weak immune systems and people with respiratory problems, it can be a killer. If you have flu, you know it. It's not just your average bad cold. My first advice is to go to bed. Don't try to keep going. It's not clever or brave. It's downright stupid and selfish. Not only are you going to make it harder for your system to recover in the long term – and getting over flu can take weeks – you're spreading all your germs to everyone else, people who maybe can't fight it off so easily. You will have guessed I don't have a lot of time for these fancy advertisements that show people walking around 24 hours after they developed flu. And I don't. Flu is an illness I respect because it's so nasty! So go to bed and rest. Drink lots of fluids and soups. Onion and/or chicken with lots of garlic is recommended. Keep warm. Keep an eye on your respiratory system to be sure that something else isn't developing. Even when you're up and on your feet after a day or two, take it easy. Don't push yourself. In the long run it's not worth it.

PREVENTION: Really very difficult. Even though flu jabs are available, the flu that's going about might be of a different type and as you can't ask it not to attack you, there's not a lot you can do. However, if you take certain immune system boosters regularly, it might cut down on the severity of the attack, or even help you miss it all together.

ECHINACEA: This one is very good for doing just that. There's quite a bit of research on it too. Not only does is boost the immune system, but it can also relieve flu symptoms. (See Echinacea, page 161.)

EUCALYPTUS: This is a good oil to burn in the sick room. You can try inhaling it too if you have flu. It certainly helps clear the tubes! (See Eucalyptus, page 164.)

GOLDENSEAL: This contains substances that activate the white blood cells, thus helping you fight flu.

ELDERBERRY: There is a patented Israeli flu drug that contains the substances found in elderberry. Since these substances also stop the virus from entering the respiratory cells, and help relieve fever, this is worth a try. Either look for teas or a tincture containing it and keep them handy if flu is on the prowl, or make a nice hot drink from the juice or wine. (See Elderberry, page 163.)

MARSH MALLOW: Marsh mallow is also fairly effective against coughs and sore throats and comes in tablet form. (See Marsh mallow, page 220.)

ZINC: I find zinc lozenges extremely effective against a sore throat, especially when taken at the outset before things get too bad. (See Zinc, page 225.)

GARLIC: Garlic capsules can help against both colds and flu and are very easy to come by. (See Garlic, page 175.)

A WORD OF CAUTION: Please refer to the individual remedy for any cautions.

INTERESTING FACT: Let's hope there's never another outbreak of Spanish flu, which stalked the land after World War I, claiming the lives of thousands in a matter of hours and caused the internal organs to disintegrate.

Freckles

Here's one for you, 'Mix together equal volumes of peroxide of hydrogen, strained lemon juice, glycerine and rosewater. With a fine, camel's hair brush apply the mixture, painting it on each individual freckle.' That's if you've got time. These well-to-do Victorian ladies certainly did – in between ordering the maid about! Seriously, that is a very old recipe, from Victorian times (although I would not recommend trying it, as hydrogen peroxide could burn your skin if not properly diluted). Apparently, too, you should 'always apply a layer of almond or olive oil to the skin before going out into the sun to protect from freckles and burning'. How times have changed. I mean, nothing about factor 6 or anything! Of course, the Victorian ladies liked their pale complexions. No doubt if you have freckles you've learned to live with them, or you couldn't care less about them. But maybe not. Or maybe you're just a summer case – someone who gets them from being in the sun. So I thought I'd include a few tips, as it were. And not just the ones above!

ELDERFLOWER, CRANBERRY, LEMON JUICE, CASTOR OIL: If you choose any two of these and mix together, then dab the mixture on your face with cotton wool, you should find that the freckles start to disappear.

HORSERADISH AND SOUR MILK: Definitely not for drinking! Mix four tablespoons of sour milk with one tablespoon of oatmeal and one teaspoon of horseradish. Then, making sure you avoid your eyes, apply the resulting paste and leave for 30 minutes. Rinse off and, hey presto, I should hope the freckles should begin to disappear.

A WORD OF CAUTION: Obviously, if your skin starts to itch, remove the preparation in case you have an allergy.

INTERESTING FACT: Fresh buttermilk was another Victorian remedy for freckles.

Fungal infections

I've looked at candida (which is one of the best-known fungal infections) in a section of its own, so what I'm doing here is simply listing some of the herbs and oils that can be used to treat any fungal infection that comes up on the body's sweaty parts: feet, toes, mouth. I'm fairly confident that these should help.

ECHINACEA: This is one for athlete's foot in particular. Just buy a tincture at your health shop and add the recommended amount to juice, twice a day. Or look for tablets. Some even come linking echinacea to another herb. If it's one listed here, then so much the better. (See Echinacea, page 161.)

GOLDENSEAL: Traditionally, goldenseal was used for just this. If you have a stubborn fungal infection that won't clear, ask at your health shop for a tincture and apply according to the instructions. Or put six teaspoons of the dried root in a cup of boiling water, simmer for 15 minutes, cool, then apply to the affected area.

MYRRH: Myrrh is very good for treating inflammation, mouth ulcers and allergies, so I'd give it a go, as some ulcers are caused by fungal infections. Ask at your health shop for capsules, cut open, then sprinkle on the infection. (See Myrrh, page 206.)

MARIGOLD: Pour boiling water over the flower heads and steep for ten minutes. Strain and apply the liquid to the affected area. Simple as pie and quite effective!

CAMOMILE: Camomile tea can be both drunk and used on the skin – oh, and bathed in – if you have a fungal infection. Just brew up a cup and either take it or apply to the affected area with a cloth. If you have hayfever you might have to find something else though. (See Camomile, page 145.)

LICORICE: Add six teaspoons of dried root to a cup of boiling water, simmer for 15 minutes, then, when it is cool, apply to the affected area. Licorice is very good for treating fungal infections generally. That's why I recommend it to my clients. (See Licorice, page 195.)

TEA TREE: This is another of my favourites for dealing with a fungal infection on the skin and foot. Just dab on a few drops of the essential oil, twice a day. It's a powerful antiseptic. Remember not to take the oil – it's poisonous. (See Tea tree oil, page 233.)

A WORD OF CAUTION: Please refer to the individual remedy you require and follow according to the instructions. Never take something that's meant for external use only.

INTERESTING FACT: Garlic was traditionally used to cure fungal infections of the feet. I would think the smell must have literally chased them away!

genital herpes

Okay, this is an embarrassing one if you're unlucky enough to have it. Certainly something you're not going to mention at supper parties without causing the person next to you to squirm on their chair, probably in the direction away from you. That's in case they get it. Herpes is actually very contagious, although common sense would tell you that it can't be spread that way. The real problem with herpes is that people actually have the virus for two or three days before the symptoms appear and sometimes they don't know they have it when they pass it on. The symptoms are tingling, burning or a persistent itch, then pimply lumps come up on the skin. These turn into blisters that burst and exude pus and blood. About a week after the first burning feeling, scabs form on the blisters and they begin to heal. At least you hope they're beginning to heal. The problem is that sometimes they reappear. It's a virus that's very difficult to get rid of in some cases.

PREVENTION: Sorry to sound like an old fuddy-duddy here but the virus that causes genital herpes is very contagious, and is mainly spread by sexual contact. So watch your partner and remember all the warnings about casual sex.

LEMON BALM: Also known as Melissa, this herb contains antioxidant vitamins. It boosts the immune system and can be effective if taken as a tea. You could then press the bags on the lesions. If you can't find it as a tea, then get the herb and add it to a cup of ordinary tea.

ECHINACEA: This is especially good for recurrent herpes. Nowadays it's very easy to come by in tablet form. It also comes as a tincture, which can be taken two or three times a day. (See Echinacea, page 161.)

GARLIC: This is useful against many viruses, so it's worth a try. Capsules are readily available. (See Garlic, page 174.)

RED PEPPER (CAYENNE POWDER): The pain-relieving qualities of red pepper are gradually being recognised. While I wouldn't recommend rubbing it on the genital area unless you want to go dancing through the roof, you could try buying it in capsule form. (See Red pepper, page 220.)

A WORD OF CAUTION: Please refer to the individual remedy for further information.

INTERESTING FACT: Well, are there any? The virus comes in two forms: cold sore and genital herpes, and is a cousin to the one that causes shingles.

Gingivitis

Gingivitis is an inflammation of the gums. It causes swelling, redness, bleeding, watery discharge, a change in the contours of the gums themselves, and dentists treat it with antiseptics. If you want something different, there are some remedies you can try. If you don't treat it, the chances are it will get worse, leading to problems, not just for your gums, but your teeth. Although sufferers can be young, it tends to strike as people get older.

PREVENTION: Like everything else, it's a case of taking care. If you look after your teeth properly, cleaning them after every meal and using floss to prevent the build up of bacteria, then you are cutting your chances of getting gingivitis. However, it can still strike. Generally, too, people who are deficient in vitamin C are more at risk of getting gum disease. So make sure there is plenty in your diet.

CAMOMILE: Camomile can help treat gingivitis, when used as a mouthwash. (See Camomile, page 145.)

EUCALYPTUS: Gum disease generally can be fought by massaging eucalyptus oil into the affected area. (See Eucalyptus, page 164.)

ECHINACEA: Adding a few drops of echinacea tincture – available from your health shop – to a camomile tea mouthwash can help fight the bacteria that cause gingivitis, and can also treat it. (See Echinacea, page 161.)

SAGE: This was a common Victorian remedy for healthy gums and white teeth. If you want to know more about how to make the tea, then see the section on sage (page 227).

PEPPERMINT: Don't think because your toothpaste says peppermint, it is anything more than peppermint flavoured. If you have a clump of this in your garden, then use the leaves. Steep three or four in a cup of boiling water for ten minutes. Then use as a mouthwash. That's the real way to take peppermint! (See Peppermint, page 215.)

NETTLE: Nettle tea can reduce and prevent gingivitis. Either ask at your health shop for dental products containing it, or try boiling the leaves in water, straining, cooling and rinsing your mouth. Don't worry, the leaves lose their sting when they are cooked! But remember to wear gloves when you first pick them! (See Nettle, page 207.)

CALENDULA: Calendula can help treat gingivitis and may even be something you've got in the garden. (See Calendula, page 144.)

A WORD OF CAUTION: Please remember to refer to the individual herb you are considering using. Hayfever sufferers, for example, may be allergic to camomile and calendula. Sage in high doses can cause convulsions.

INTERESTING FACT: The Chinese chew watercress to keep their gums healthy.

Gout

Gout is a constitutional disorder connected with an excess of uric acid in the blood. The joint, not only becomes inflamed, but extremely painful and tender. Usually it affects the big toe and strikes without warning, overnight, leaving the poor sufferer unable to walk, in many cases. Since those who are overweight or have high blood pressure are more at risk of developing it, changes to the diet can certainly help to treat it, as can losing weight. But please do this sensibly and slowly. Taking too much off too quickly achieves nothing. Avoiding alcohol can also help. If you are a sufferer and don't want to stop drinking entirely – a dire thought for anyone! – then limit your intake. This can certainly reduce the number of attacks. Changes to the diet can include avoiding sweetbreads, red meat, chicken, turkey, sardines and herring. Looking at the list of what to avoid makes me wonder what's left. Certainly there's fresh vegetables and fruit – again a tall order. So try to limit the intake of certain things, which in turn should reduce the number of attacks you suffer.

CHERRY JUICE: For years it has been thought that cherry juice helps reduce the pain and inflammation caused by gout, although the actual reason for this remains unclear. Many sufferers swear by it however, so you could try making cherries a vital part of your diet if you're a sufferer, either canned or fresh, or as a juice. You can even make your own if you have a liquidiser.

PINEAPPLE: Pineapples contain a substance that helps break down protein, so this is another good fruit to start including in your diet.

VITAMIN C: This has been shown to rid the body of uric acid. Either eat more fruit regularly, thus ensuring your body has enough, or take a supplement.

CELERY: Celery also helps eliminate uric acid. (See Celery, page 148.)

QUERCETIN: You could try taking quercetin tablets, available from your health shop. Quercetin is known to stop the growth of the enzyme that produces uric acid.

OLIVE: Since all the old medical books talk of purging the system to flush out the uric acids, you might like to give olive, a try, or indeed any diuretic herb or fruit. The use of olives is this respect goes back to biblical times. If you don't like them, fine. Any herb or fruit that has a diuretic affect will be helpful during an attack. The only down side is you'll have to keep hobbling to the loo!

AVAILABILITY: Cherries, pineapples and olives can be easily come by. If you don't like eating them fresh, try drinking the juice. Vitamin C is available in tablet form, or as a refreshing drink, from supermarkets or health shops. Quercetin is available from the latter.

INTERESTING FACT: Historically, gout was known as the rich man's disease. The poor man was probably just as likely to get it. He just wasn't able to indulge it!

Haemorrhoids

Here's another one nobody likes to talk about. Although I've a sneaking suspicion that if you're looking up this section you know exactly what they are and you don't need me to tell you about the pain! For those who aren't certain, haemorrhoids (also known as 'piles' – as in: 'My piles are giving me gyp!') are enlarged veins in the anus or rectum. From time to time they can bleed and become painful and itchy enough to drive the sufferer insane. And, of course, being where they are, well, you can't go around scratching, now can you? You also worry about going to the toilet. So what do you do? Well the best way to deal with haemorrhoids is to prevent them. And that goes for those who have them too. Unless of course yours are very severe. In which case you're probably waiting for surgery!

PREVENTION: Well, first of all you need to be sure, in terms of the bleeding, that what you have are haemorrhoids. And usually it is. So don't go off panic-stricken at this point thinking you've got something worse! If these symptoms are present then it's likely that this is what you've got. However, any unusual or unexplained bleeding should be investigated, which means putting your embarrassment aside and seeing a doctor. Most doctors think that haemorrhoids are caused by constipation, although, conversely, some can be caused by diarrhoea. In some instances among pregnant women, haemorrhoids can be caused by the pressure of the foetus on the veins of the leg. In order to prevent haemorrhoids you have to prevent constipation and keep the body functioning regularly. Eating lots of fruit and vegetables can help. Ones that are especially good are apples and carrots. You should also try to include cereals such as bran. Drink lots of water. Fresh orange juice is also good. These act as 'lubricants', preventing irritation in that very vital area when you do visit the bathroom. Talking of visiting the bathroom, straining just makes things worse. Even if you don't have haemorrhoids, don't strain – children are sometimes very guilty of this, if the sounds coming out the bathroom are anything to go by! Rather, take something that is mildly laxative and wait. Also, never ignore the 'urge to go'. That just causes things to 'pile on the pile', so to speak! For more advice on diet and constipation please look at the section on constipation (pages 35–8), and also the one on bran (pages 137–8). In this section what I'm going to cover now is what to do to treat the haemorrhoid itself.

WITCH HAZEL: This is a soothing astringent which can help itching and also pain. Just apply with cotton wool or put a little on a piece of linen and tuck in place. (See Witch hazel, page 252.)

COMFREY: Comfrey has anti-inflammatory compounds, making it useful for relieving pain and swelling. Either make a compress with some tincture in water, or if you have the plant itself, pound the leaf and rub it carefully on. (See Comfrey, page 154.)

ALOE VERA: The gel itself can be used to calm the haemorrhoid down, while the juice can be drunk for a laxative effect. Just take 2–3 glasses a day until the problem has cleared. (See Aloe Vera, page 121.)

BUTCHER'S BROOM: This herb is good for varicose veins and that's what haemorrhoids are. Either look for a tincture and apply as described above or make a tea by placing four teaspoonfuls in boiling water, steeping for 20 minutes, then drinking. If you don't like the taste, add honey.

A WORD OF CAUTION: As I said above, if you are experiencing bleeding which doesn't seem to relate to haemorrhoids, please see a doctor for your own sake. Refer to the individual remedy that you choose to be sure it is suitable for you. Never take anything that is meant for external use only.

INTERESTING FACT: While we might not like to talk about it and estimates vary, it is thought that up to one in three people do, or will, have the joy of experiencing haemorrhoids at some time in their life.

Halitosis

Here's one nobody likes much and I can't say I blame them. Putting somebody 'off' with the smell of our breath is something we all dread. And let's be absolutely honest here, how many of us have mouths that smell like daisies when we get up in the morning? No matter how careful we are during the day about cleaning and rinsing and flossing, the salivary glands slow at night. Sometimes, too, we eat something that isn't so nice for the mouth when we're in a situation where we can't clean or floss or rinse. When the mouth dries, too, often in a stressful situation, halitosis can strike. It certainly loves us, though we don't care for it. Can we do something?

PREVENTION: Cleaning and flossing regularly help keep the mouth clean and generally bacteria-free. So does using mouthwashes. But bad breath can sometimes be a sign of something more serious. If it is very bad and shows no sign of clearing with anything at all, please see your doctor.

EUCALYPTUS: Using a mouthwash with a drop of eucalyptus oil can certainly help bad breath. (See Eucalyptus, page 164.)

PARSLEY: Parsley is very good for freshening the breath. If you can't clean your teeth and there's some parsley on the salad, there's your answer.

SAGE: You can try making a mouthwash with sage tea. It's very good for the health of the gums in general. (See Sage, page 227.)

PEPPERMINT: I would recommend rinsing with peppermint tea rather than the oil, as the latter is particularly toxic when swallowed. Also, it's always handy to keep a packet of mints in your bag or pocket. If you're eating out or your mouth dries, then they can at least keep it fresh and smelling pleasant till you can clean your teeth properly.

A WORD OF CAUTION: Please refer to individual herbs before you start trying them. Some have side effects, while others are toxic if swallowed.

INTERESTING FACT: She may have looked as if she was enjoying every minute of Clark Gable's company in *Gone with the Wind*, but Vivian Leigh was so sick of the smell of his dentures that tomorrow nearly wasn't another day at all. She refused to film any more love scenes unless he did something about it.

Hangover

What is 'hangover' doing in a health book I hear you say? Well, let's be honest, alternative medicine isn't all about being super-healthy, herb-eating gurus, wandering about the bushes in search of our Ylang Ylang. It's about finding other ways of doing things, trying to benefit conditions we may already have, knowing what to do if we haven't got conventional medicine to hand, or conventional medicine doesn't seem to be helping, and it's also about eating to keep healthy. Okay, so some of us drink too! We can't all be paragons of virtue! And sometimes we drink a little too much! Sometimes we don't even need to be drunk, or drink too much, to experience a hangover, either. For certain people, two glasses of wine can be too much, for others that's just an aperitif! Hangovers can sometimes come about because we're run down generally or about to develop an illness. You know the 'I didn't drink any more than I usually do' feeling you experience as you lie with your head down the toilet bowl. Generally, however, hangovers do come about because we've drunk too much. I don't think I really need to go through the symptoms here, but basically they include headache, muscle ache, vomiting and feeling like you're going to die.

PREVENTION: Well that's fairly obvious really. Don't drink – don't get hungover. But that's very difficult to do. So be realistic. Don't mix drinks. Stick to white-coloured drinks rather than dark ones. Try alternating your drinks with water. Eat as you drink to mop up the alcohol. Don't drink on an empty stomach – you really will get drunk much faster, and hungover too. Put a good lining, such as milk, on the stomach before you go out. When you come in, drink a good two tumblers of water. 'Up all night, then, in the loo?' – I don't think so. Alcohol dehydrates. That's the main reason for a hangover. You may ask how I know all this. I won't say!

GINGKO BILOBA: Gets a good name for a hangover, as it clears the alcohol from the blood. So you can try taking some the morning after, so to speak. I don't want to say before you go out. It may only encourage you! (See Gingko biloba, page 177.)

WINTERGREEN: The herbal aspirin should soothe the sore head and shivering limbs. But if you're allergic to aspirin, you'll be allergic to this too, so please take note and follow the instructions. (See Wintergreen, page 250.)

HONEY: There are as many hangover remedies as there are hangovers. Everyone has their own favourite. I don't. Not because I don't drink. If I have a hangover, I'm just too ill to think of one! This is one that comes up repeatedly, so I think it's worth a try. Put a teaspoon in a cup of tea. (That's providing you can drink tea!)

GINGER: Ginger does help nausea, so perhaps adding some to a cup of tea might help. (See Ginger, page 175.)

PEPPERMINT: Peppermint tea can stop the spasms that cause retching. That's assuming you're not retching so much you can't get anything down. If you can, then try this to stop the nausea. (See Peppermint, page 215.)

INTERESTING FACT: The Japanese actually serve gingko seeds at parties to cut down on drunkenness.

Headache

Now, unless we've all been living on the planet Zog, we all know what this is, so I'm not going to describe it in any detail. Migraine is already covered elsewhere (page 88). What I'm looking at here are just plain old headaches and plain old cures.

PREVENTION: Many headaches are caused by stress, being too long in the sun and not drinking enough. The latter two types are certainly quite preventable if you take care, when sunbathing or out in the heat, to make sure you drink plenty of fluids constantly – soft drinks, that is, not alcoholic ones. What a spoilsport, eh! You should also wear a hat. Stress headaches can be helped by cutting down on the stress. Look at the way you are living. Are there changes you can make? Do you eat regularly and properly? That kind of thing. Other headaches can be caused by colds, flu or periods. For all of them you might find these remedies useful.

WILLOW: Willow bark is the herbal aspirin. In fact it was the first aspirin, if you like. I'd recommend it for all types of headache mentioned above, provided you follow the instructions.

EVENING PRIMROSE OIL: This contains many pain-relieving compounds. If you are a woman and your headache is linked to 'that time of the month' then you might find it useful to take it over the course of your period, even starting a few days before. (See Evening primrose oil, page 165.)

CAMOMILE: This is the one I recommend for stress. A cup of tea if you have a headache is very soothing. (See Camomile, page 145.)

PEPPERMINT/LAVENDER: Rubbing peppermint or lavender oil on the temples can be very effective for a headache.

LEMON BALM AND GINGER: A tea made with lemon balm and a little ginger can also be very good for relieving a sore head. Or look in your health shop to see if you can buy one.

GARLIC: This one's good for a headache caused by cold or flu. You can either take capsules or add it to your food. (See Garlic, page 174.)

ELDERBERRY: Elderberry is also good for colds and flu and cold-induced headaches. (See Elderberry, page 163.)

A WORD OF CAUTION: Please refer to the individual remedy you choose for information on any cautions.

INTERESTING FACT: Bay was traditionally used to cure a headache.

Immune system

Having a healthy immune system is so important it's hardly worth stating here. When the immune system is weak, all kinds of infections and viruses strike. That's why often when we have one illness such as flu, another comes at the back, leaving us feeling even worse. Then there's the long fight, or so it seems anyway, back to feeling fully fit again. Sometimes people don't. That's when conditions such as chronic fatigue can strike. There are other things, too, that can go wrong with the immune system. Viruses that won't go away, largely because they've knocked out our immunity and are having a perfectly nice time where they are – even thinking of sending you a postcard, so to speak. We all know, too, of the terrible havoc being wreaked by AIDS. Herbs can't cure it. I'm not going to pretend. That would be pointless and wrong of me. But I don't think we can pretend it doesn't exist, either. What I'm doing here is simply listing the herbs and foodstuffs that can help promote a healthy immune system generally.

DIET: Like everything else, diet has its part to play in keeping the immune system healthy and functioning to the best of its ability. The foodstuffs to include if you're feeling under par, or want to tone up the system generally are: onions, garlic, ginger, pears, elderberry and oregano. They are the best things when it comes to giving the system what it needs. Generally, eating lots of fruit and vegetables helps, too. That's what I've always been told anyhow and I've no reason not to believe it! Vitamins can also help – vitamins C and B12, as well as E.

ECHINACEA: This has long been regarded as an antiviral herb, ideal for boosting the immune system to fight viruses. One of the substances in it actually boosts the white blood cells across the body. It's very easy to find and take, coming as a capsule, often combined with other immune boosters, or a tincture. (See Echinacea, page 161.)

BURDOCK: Traditionally very good for fighting viral infections. (See Burdock, page 140.)

GOLDENSEAL: Combined with echinacea, this is very good for keeping the immune system in good working order. If you have a viral infection it's worth giving it a try.

LEMON BALM: This herb is good against herpes. It also makes a pleasant tea.

LICORICE: This contains so many compounds it would take me all day to list them. And as I haven't got that, I'm just going to say that one of them helps stop viral infections blooming and taking over. Ask at your health shop for supplements, or make a tea by steeping a teaspoon of the chopped dried root in a cup of boiling water. (See Licorice, page 195.)

KOREAN GINSENG: This helps strengthen the immune system generally. (See Ginseng – Asian, page 179.)

GINGKO BILOBA: This is one of my favourites. It's good for a great many things and boosting the immune system is one of them. (See Gingko biloba, page 177.)

A WORD OF CAUTION: Please remember to refer to the individual supplement for any herbal remedy that you choose. If you have a serious health worry, something that's not really clearing, see your doctor. If you're none the wiser as to what it is, then at least you know what it's not!

INTERESTING FACT: Research is ongoing into the anti-viral properties in St John's Wort.

Indigestion

Here's one we all know well, brought about by heaping too much food on our poor systems. Christmas dinners are fatal, let's be honest! So I'm not going to go into all the symptoms. If you're reading this, then you know! You're looking for a remedy, not me 'bag of winding on'. So here goes.

PREVENTION: Well that's obvious isn't it? Don't overeat. But some indigestion is caused by certain foods. If there's something that seems to torture your system, then stay off it. Rich fatty foods are worst. When you're cooking a large meal, try adding certain things that will help – they're listed below, as well as some other remedies. That way you shouldn't suffer so much. Excessive acid is the main cause of indigestion. Eat regularly rather than bingeing all at once. And eat small meals where possible. Also, take your time. Bolting back the mouthfuls creates wind and other digestive discomforts.

CAMOMILE: This is one of my favourites for stomach problems. It's a gentle relaxant and so soothing for the system. If you're having a dinner party or serving any kind of large meal, this is actually much better than coffee to finish off with. (See Camomile, page 145.)

PEPPERMINT: Again, ending a large meal with a nice cup of peppermint tea is a good way of ensuring that your guests don't suffer from excess! People might look at you to start with, but they'll soon thank you when they don't suffer for the rest of the evening. You might even start a trend! I also use it when someone has indigestion. It soon seems to settle things down. (See Peppermint, page 215.)

GINGER: Another of my 'tricks' is just to put a half-teaspoon of ginger in a cup of tea. It may taste a bit odd but it aids the digestion by moving the food through the intestine. Or you can try smelling the oil. (See Ginger, page 175.)

LAVENDER, JUNIPER, BASIL, ROSEMARY: All these oils are very good for indigestion. Keep a little bottle of any of them handy and sniff if you're suffering. Remember not to take the oil.

BLESSED THISTLE: This herb is good for easing a bout of indigestion. Ask at your health shop and keep handy.

WILD YAM: I'm not talking about the vegetable here but the tablets you can buy at any health shop. They're very good for many digestive problems, indigestion being only one.

RED PEPPER (CAYENNE POWDER): Now I'm coming to the spices and herbs to add to food to help in their digestion and, contrary to what many people believe, red pepper is one. Although hot and spicy, it stimulates the digestion, so sprinkling a little into the rice or pasta or even vegetables you're preparing is a good idea.

SAGE, BASIL, CORIANDER, CINNAMON, OREGANO, ROSEMARY, CHIVES, CLOVES, DILL: These are also excellent when put in food in advance.

PARSLEY: Keeping a piece of parsley handy and saving it till last not only freshens the breath but helps the digestion. (See Parsley, page 213.)

A WORD OF CAUTION: Please refer to the individual remedies you choose to use. Continual indigestion can be the sign of other stomach problems. Please see a doctor if it is worrying you.

Infertility

Infertility is generally defined by doctors as the failure to become pregnant after a year of unprotected intercourse. And, however it's defined, it is a big heartache for those who find themselves in this position. The possible cause should always be diagnosed by a doctor first and before you go getting depressed about it, and thinking 'Oh, I'll never have a baby,' some of the reasons for infertility are quite sortable. Where women are concerned, it might be there is a problem with the tubes that requires a little surgery and, in instances like this, all the herbal remedies and dietary changes in the world won't make any difference. Sometimes, however, other things are at fault – low sperm counts, or just what seems to be no reason at all. This is what I'm trying to look at here.

LIFESTYLE: Some studies link smoking and drinking to a failure to conceive where women are concerned. I do stress the word, 'some'. Obviously plenty people do both and have no trouble conceiving. Women who are overweight or underweight can also find it harder to conceive and in some instances certain medicines can also cause infertility.

DIET: Caffeine has been shown to reduce female fertility. Again, this doesn't hold good for everyone and no doubt there are other reasons you can't conceive that have nothing to with how many cups of coffee you drink a day. But some studies do show that as little as one cup of coffee a day can delay conception. So maybe you should cut out the coffee, cocoa and hot chocolate. Nutritional deficiencies can lead to infertility for both sexes. If you've got a sort of 'unexplained infertility', or a low sperm count, it does no harm to up your intake of spinach, cauliflower, broccoli, peas and onions. In addition to this, you men should think about adding some ginger, fenugreek, chives and red pepper to your food and eating plenty Brazil nuts, peanuts, almonds – oh, and oats! While that may make you sound a bit like a horse, and induce jokes about randy stallions, there is some truth in the old saying. Oats do increase male fertility, while the others are good for low sperm counts. Other herbs and supplements include:

VITAMIN E: A preliminary trial indicates that taking vitamin E can increase fertility in both men and women.

GINSENG: Ginseng has been used for hundreds of years to increase male potency in Asia, so there's no harm in having a go. (See Ginseng, page 179.)

A WORD OF CAUTION: Don't despair. It's very important that you don't blame each other. Try to find some inner peace about the matter.

INTERESTING FACT: Infertility must be the subject of more old wives' tales than most. 'Doing it with your boots on' is but one!

Insect bites

Insect bites are great fun – of course I'm joking! From the common old midge in Britain, to the mosquitoes of more exotic climes, don't these little things just love to make our lives a misery! Fleas too! The world is full of them! Most of us know the signs – red spots. The size and kind of spot may vary according to the insect. Mosquito bites for example come up in large watery-looking blisters. Bite pens or sticks for dealing with bites are now widely available but there are also some herbal remedies you can try.

PREVENTION: Really very difficult. Hill walkers and mountain climbers curse the midges. Foreign travellers, the mosquito. And some people tend to suffer more than others. Wearing a repellent can help, either driving the insects away or at least cutting down the amount that attack. Midges like the places with dense undergrowth. Make sure you cover up, unless you want to be chewed alive. With regard to mosquitoes, they tend to attack more at night, when their blood lust is at its most desperate. If you're applying a repellent then make sure your ankles and legs are covered. That's the area they love making a tasty meal of, while you're tucking into yours. Also make sure that you deal with mosquito bites. Sometimes they become infected, then the whole area swells. If that happens, keep applying an antiseptic cream and ice-packs. Seek medical advice if it shows no sign of getting better, or indeed worsens. It may be you need some anti-histamine tablets and if you do, you do. Remember alternative medicine isn't about becoming a martyr because you want to do things the natural way. It's about using your sense to judge what is right and what is wrong for you.

CITRUS OIL: This is a good repellent. Generally, insects don't like the smell of citrus fruits. Either wear a citrus perfume, or dilute some oil in vegetable oil and smear it on.

BASIL: Basil is also good for driving the insects away. In some countries the leaves are just rubbed on the skin.

TEA TREE OIL: Some people swear by this and now, in addition to the oil, there are a great many beauty care products containing it. I would, however, recommend buying the oil and dabbing it on. Bugs seem to loathe it! Tea tree is also good if you are bitten. (See Tea tree oil, page 233.)

CALENDULA: Cream containing calendula is very effective against insect bites. The flowers, too, but I'm saying cream here because if you've just been bitten, the chances are you don't want to trail round looking for calendula flowers! It may be winter after all! (See Calendula, page 144.)

GARLIC: Garlic helps reduce inflammation and can be swallowed or applied. Taking capsules while you're on holiday may, for example, help cut down the risk of infection if you are bitten. As well as eating garlic, you can apply it to the bite as a poultice. (See Garlic, page 174.)

ONION: Because they contain quercetin, onions can help reduce bite inflammation. The skins are best and should be boiled for ten minutes. Once the liquid has cooled, dab it on the bite. As well as relieving the inflammation, the liquid from boiled onion skins can stop itching. I know, I've tried it! (See Onion, page 210.)

A WORD OF CAUTION: Please refer to the individual herb for any side effects. Calendula, for example, can sometimes irritate hayfever sufferers.

INTERESTING FACT: Pennyroyal was used hundreds of years ago as an insect repellent.

Insomnia

Insomnia – the inability to fall asleep or stay asleep – can affect us all at some time in our lives. Often the cause is stress, over-tiredness (funnily enough), illness or an upset to our normal sleep routines, which then sends our body clock haywire and makes it hard to get back to normal. But it's not funny when this happens. Going to bed becomes a worry because we know we're going to lie awake another night. However, there are some solutions we can try that will hopefully help. Some of these involve herbal medicines. Others are common sense, although that's hard to see when we're tired and irritable. I'm going to look at these first, then at the herbals. You can see if there's something there for you.

STRESS: Many of us lead busy lives then expect to fall into bed at night and get to sleep instantly. If you take your day to bed with you, so to speak, you won't sleep well. Try to wind down at bedtime: read, take a herbal bath (see Lavender, page 192), or a cup of camomile tea. If you have problems and worries, things to attend to the next day, for example, make a list. If there's been an argument with a close partner, try to resolve it. Remember the saying, 'never let the sun go down on your anger'. Well, I don't know the next bit but it should be, 'or you won't get a good night's sleep', because you won't. If your mind is racing, try lying on your back for a while and imagining you are somewhere really nice, a place you want to be. Block out everything else except the details of this place and how calm and soothing it is.

EXERCISE: If you're active during the day, you'll sleep better at night. Only don't be too active. The secret is to achieve a happy medium. If you do too much, you'll be too tired to sleep. And don't do something like going for a jog just before you turn in. The best time for exercise is before 7 p.m. Obviously, if you don't do much during the day you won't sleep at night. So don't expect to. Sometimes the body just takes what it needs.

ILLNESS: If you have an injury that keeps you awake, or if you are ill, then you won't sleep as much as usual. No matter how tempting it is to lie in bed, dosing off and on all morning, try to wake up early. You don't have to get up if you can't. Just stay awake, and try to do so most of the day, going to sleep at your usual time. Sleeping late in the morning adds to the problem, because it sets the body off on a different 'clock' altogether – a bit like jet lag.

VALERIAN: Valerian is good for insomnia and relaxation in general (See Valerian, page 239.)

CAMOMILE: This is one I like. While it doesn't send you 'out like a light', it does help you relax, especially when taken before a herbal bath. This is because it contains a sedative compound. (See Camomile, page 145.)

LAVENDER: Lavender oil is used by many aromatherapists and can definitely help reduce restlessness. It's another favourite of mine. (See Lavender, page 192.)

A WORD OF CAUTION: Remember to give whichever remedy you choose time to work. It may be that drinking camomile, for example, throughout the day has a relaxing effect and when bedtime comes you've no trouble getting off to sleep. Also, remember not to take things every single night. The remedies mentioned are not addictive but obviously it's best at times to fall asleep naturally if you can.

INTERESTING FACT: Sleep problems may be genetic. Present research indicates that a single gene is responsible for the body's internal clock. Counting sheep irritates me and, if anything, makes me more awake, especially when I lose count. I personally prefer to 'spend' my make-believe win on the lottery. At least I fall asleep happy!

Irritable bowel syndrome

Irritable Bowel Syndrome (IBS) is more a discomfort than a serious health threat. That's all very well for me to say, I hear you muttering! But if I recommend something to help, I'm sure you'll forgive me! The symptoms include, bloating, wind, soreness, alternating constipation and diarrhoea and, in some instances, sore back, headache and fatigue. Quite a lot really! The actual cause isn't known, although I would hazard a little guess that diet and nutrition probably plays its part, maybe not even in the way you would suspect, i.e. 'I eat a lot of rubbish.' So let's look there first.

DIET: Some cases are actually caused by food allergies. The stomach just doesn't like what you're putting in it. If you can take note of what these are by keeping a record of attacks and what you ate, then you might be able to identify the problem foods and avoid them. Obviously they're different for everyone, so I can't make a full list here, although I can say that some people can't absorb lactose (milk and dairy products), fructose (fruit juice and dried fruit) and sorbitol (certain sweets). Looking at this list, it's safe to say that although you might be making an effort to eat healthy foods, in your case, sadly, some of them aren't helping. If you suffer from constipation too, you've maybe been trying things like bran to help. If you have an allergy to wheat, it won't help. Try brown rice, oatmeal and psyllium husks instead. However, if you're diabetic, avoid the latter, as it contains sugar.

CAMOMILE: Sometimes stress plays a big part in triggering attacks of this condition. Camomile tea or tincture could be helpful in this case. Not only does it act as a gentle relaxant but it helps tone the stomach muscles and soothe cramps. (See Camomile, page 145.)

PEPPERMINT: Peppermint is also good for calming the stomach and getting rid of wind. Either finish your meals with a cup of peppermint tea or look for capsules at your health shop.

FENNEL: Fennel generally aids the digestive tract and has few side effects. (See Fennel, page 167.)

EVENING PRIMROSE OIL: Some women only experience IBS before or during their period, while some report a worsening of the condition. If this sounds like you, try evening primrose oil before your period is due. It's excellent for regulating everything and helping with the conditions associated with menstruation. (See Evening primrose oil, page 165.)

PSYLLIUM: Though you must avoid these husks if you're diabetic, psyllium seeds or husks stimulate the bowel. You can also buy capsules.

A WORD OF CAUTION: Please refer to individual references for remedies for any cautions.

INTERESTING FACT: Charlemagne grew fennel because of its healing qualities.

Itching

Itching can be caused by many things. Candida, for example, causes itching in a very sensitive place! But you'll find I've covered this elsewhere! Scabies, too, another condition that causes scratching, can be found in the appropriate section. What it is and how to deal with it, that is! I should certainly hope such a condition won't leap off these pages! What I'm going to look at here is just general skin irritation, the kind we all get from time to time, perhaps because we're allergic to something, or have been bitten, or the kind we just 'have'! Because, let's face it, once we have it, we can't stop!

PREVENTION: If you seem to be allergic to a particular substance, then the answer is simple. Try to find out first of all what it is and stop using it. Some itches, too, start from wearing clothes that are too tight on certain parts of the body and are setting up a moisture rash. Some woollen fabrics just naturally seem to cause an itch. The real problem with an itch is scratching, because then the skin breaks and bleeds. Some skin problems are very hard to heal once this cycle starts. Don't neglect things to begin with. Also, please remember that severe itching in certain parts of the body can be related to a particular condition. For example, head lice result in the scalp being constantly itchy, as does dandruff. So it's important that you treat these appropriately.

ONION: I'm a great believer in boiled onion skins to soothe irritated skin and relieve general itching associated with minor skin conditions. Boil the skins for ten minutes in water, then apply the liquid to the affected area. Talk about skins for skins! (See Onion, page 210.)

CALENDULA: This is very good for soothing itchy skin. What's more, it comes as a cream. Ask at your health shop. (See Calendula, page 144.)

WITCH HAZEL: Witch hazel is another favourite of mine. Sometimes I also use it with camomile. When I do, I make some camomile tea, pour in a little witch hazel and dab it on the itchy area. Please note, I didn't say drink it. This is one for external use only. Witch hazel can be bought in supermarkets or health shops and applied according to the instructions. (See Witch hazel, page 252.)

CAMOMILE: Gentle relaxing camomile can help itchy skin do just that. You can even try squeezing the tea bag on the affected area. (See Camomile, page 145.)

A WORD OF CAUTION: Please note these are remedies for the more minor skin conditions. Ones that nevertheless can cause very irritating itches. Please refer to Candida, Lice, Dermatitis, Scabies if you think you have something more. Also refer to the individual herbal remedy for usage instructions as some are not suitable if you have certain conditions.

INTERESTING FACT: Calamine lotion was the great unsung hero in the war against itches in the first part of the last century.

Laryngitis

Shout a lot? Sing badly? Sing at all? Speak a lot, even? Well, you may be a sufferer from this ailment – a condition that causes hoarseness or loss of voice, or both. Laryngitis is an inflammation of the vocal chords, also resulting in an unpleasant dry feeling in the throat. In some instances, because the sufferer is using their voice a lot, it can be very difficult to get rid of. In some cases, too, it is recurring. If you suffer and want a herbal remedy, here's what to do. Remember, though, that if you have chronic laryngitis you should see your doctor first, to be sure that's what it is. Sometimes chronic laryngitis can be the sign of something more serious.

PREVENTION: This can be very difficult if you use your voice a lot and are struck by a bout, especially in the typical British climate, where cold and damp are also part of the equation. Sometimes laryngitis develops after a cold, flu or bronchitis, because the throat becomes inflamed by coughing. Although this is easier said than done, try not to neglect the cough if you're suffering from these conditions and try to make sure that you treat it from the start. That way you're lessening your chances of developing this condition.

ECHINACEA: According to some studies, echinacea is good for relieving and treating laryngitis. Sometimes it can make the tongue tingle or go numb and if it does, don't worry. In addition to treating this condition, echinacea can boost the immune system, helping to fight the virus that causes it. Ask at your health shop. It may be that taking it regularly could help if you suffer repeatedly. (See Echinacea, page 161.)

IVY: Ivy is good at relieving inflammation, especially of the respiratory tract, and can help to prevent a cough. Ask at your health shop for preparations containing it. (See Ivy, page 190.)

MARSH MALLOW: Marsh mallow contains a substance that is good for throat inflammation. (See Marsh mallow, page 200.)

NETTLE: When it's boiled, nettle loses it sting. The same goes for a sore throat that nettle touches. Well, not quite! But nettle can help treat other conditions of the respiratory tract, so it's always worth a try. Put a handful of leaves in boiling water, leave to stand for ten minutes, strain, then either gargle or drink. Remember to use gloves when you pick the nettle. Ask at your health shop for tea or other products containing it, if you're worried about stings! (See Nettle, page 207.)

A WORD OF CAUTION: Please always study the instructions on any herb you are trying and if you seem allergic, discontinue use.

Herbal medicine has been used for thousands of years but it has to be used wisely.

INTERESTING FACT: Marsh Mallow has been used for thousands of years to help throat conditions.

Libido loss (both sexes)

Okay, so in many ways this can be a bit of a joke. As a culture, we are obsessed with sex. Steamy scenes in films, erotic scenes in books, advertisements that adhere to the slogan 'sex sells', jokes, exotic underwear – you'd really think no one had a problem. Unfortunately, that isn't always the case. After all, even the hottest fire can grow cold! Both men and women can go through phases where they lose interest in sex and if you're not bothered about it, fine, turn the page and move on. But many do worry about it and, in some instances, the bedroom can almost become a battlefield. In others, you're trying so desperately to enjoy yourself that it doesn't work either. So here are some hints. Some are even old folk remedies. You see, there's nothing new about this problem! It's as old as the hills! That we haven't got rid of this problem is down to some very human factors.

PREVENTION: Sorry, I'm not going to say run and buy a rather rude magazine here. Instead I'm going to talk about the factors that can cause loss of interest. I think it's important that you acknowledge the fact that there might be one there you recognise. We're very good at pushing our bodies to do all kinds of things. Sometimes when we've lost interest it's because our bodies are telling us something. Stress is a very high factor in loss of interest in sex. Let's be honest, do you really feel like it when you've been dashing around all day, seeing to lots of different things, perhaps dealing with various crises, or suffering emotional upset? I would think only a very silly person would answer 'yes'. Many women who lose interest are those with young children, who are dealing with all the demands that involves. The last thing they feel like when they get into bed is a passionate embrace. Men and women, too, who have difficult, high-stress occupations, sometimes find themselves in this category. Worries over money, employment, family, make it very difficult to switch off. Alcohol and illness are other factors. Certain medications, especially depressants, can have an effect. If you find yourself in these categories, then you might need to think about treating the bigger picture, so to speak.

If there's a problem then it's important, as a couple, that you acknowledge it. It's also important that you spend time as a couple, being just that. Sometimes, even just a relaxing change of scene for one night can make a difference, especially if you have young children, or a busy job. Having said that, some relationships have already gone so far down the road of 'no return', the old magic isn't going to come back, no matter how you try. I also think that if you've got a huge emotional crisis in your life then you should try to accept, as a couple, that one of you just doesn't feel like it and take the 'I can wait' approach, and do so, rather than trying to 'squeeze blood out a stone', so to speak. That may sound a little old fashioned, and it may not be what you want to hear, but things won't improve if you don't, and you're just creating another problem on top of the one you've got. Relaxation is also a big part of being interested in sex – if you're tense you won't be. A nice, candlelit bath in some soothing lavender might help do that. Just don't set the house on fire instead of yourself. Oh, and keep a sense of humour. That's not always easy but, if you can, keep things light and jokey, it's much easier to handle if things don't work out.

GINSENG: This is generally regarded as an aphrodisiac for both sexes. But, like many other remedies, it can be expensive, so it depends how much you want to sort out your problem! If you do, ask at your health shop and take according to the instructions.

FENUGREEK: This is good for menopausal women who may have lost interest or who perhaps find sex difficult because of vaginal dryness. Traditionally, this herb was used to make women more buxom. It has oestrogen-like compounds, so it's well worth trying.

PARSLEY: This is also one that is supposed to work for women only. It has a long history of treating female ailments. My advice would be to eat lots.

FENNEL: Fennel can be used by women, hopefully with some result. Like Fenugreek, it contains hormone-like compounds, which could increase your desire. Look for drinks containing it at your health shop. While this is safe, the extracted oil can cause miscarriage if you're pregnant, and is actually quite toxic generally, so please don't use that.

DAMIANA: Some people of both sexes swear by this herb for improving their interest in sex. Others say it does nothing for them in that regard. But then everyone's different and I can see no reason not to give it a try. (See Damiana, page 158.)

OATS: If you're a man and have lost interest because you're having problems in 'keeping things going', shall we say, then you could try oats. Steep a tablespoonful in a cup of boiling water, with a teaspoon of Damiana, cool, then drink. Or just eat lots of porridge!

GINGKO BILOBA: Gingko improves blood flow generally, throughout the body. It might well improve the blood flow to one particular organ, you never know! The only problem is that you would probably have to give it time to work. Four months is a long time to wait, I'd say! But if you have a problem maintaining an erection, then you'll be prepared to give it time to work, because it's a problem you'd like to be rid of. (See Gingko biloba, page 177.)

MASSAGE: Massage can also help a flagging sex life and, let's face it, sometimes part of the problem is we're so used to our partners. Pay a visit to the shops selling aromatherapy oils. The ones to look out for are jasmine, rose and Ylang Ylang. But so many shops now sell kits containing sensual oils, it saves a lot of trouble. Then come home, light the candles, set the scene and you might find the fire's not so cold after all. Massage is a very sensual thing, even without the oils.

VALERIAN: This is a relaxant. If stress, nervousness, or even fear, are causes of why you've gone off sex, then using valerian will help you to relax enough to at least be willing to give it a try. (See Valerian, page 239.)

A WORD OF CAUTION: Please refer to the individual reference for the remedy that interests you. Never take oils. Doing so won't improve your sex life as many are highly toxic. What it could mean is you've no life at all!

INTERESTING FACT: Bear in mind that being relaxed is of paramount importance when having sex (even more important than being 'needy', because without one you don't have the other), so use any method you personally feel comfortable with to ensure you gain some measure of relaxation.

Lice

Now we come to a condition that nobody much wants to talk about, very often because they feel ashamed. Don't be. Right at the start I'm going to say that lice like the cleanest of heads. They are also spread amongst people who know each other well. So if one member of the family is unfortunate enough to have them, you will have to think in terms of treating every member for the treatment to be at all effective. People with short hair are more easily infected, whilst those with long hair find it hardest to cure. The most common symptom of lice is excessive itching, although that is not always the case. Sometimes there are no symptoms at all, so you then have to know what to look for. Stand over a sink or basin of water and comb your hair with a fine-toothed comb, available from all chemists, making long, firm strokes from the scalp to the tips. Stop between each stroke to dip the comb in water. Actual lice are about the size of a match head. They are wingless and grey in colour. The eggs, 'nits', are the little white gluey specks that look like dandruff, only they don't ping away as dandruff does. They cling.

REASSURANCE: Children in particular feel ashamed if they find they have this infection, so if this is the case reassure your child that they are in no way to blame – it does not mean that their personal hygiene is not up to standard.

KWELL SHAMPOO: This is available from chemists and, used according to the instructions, will bring the problem under control.

DETECTION COMBING: Don't just treat the head and assume that's that. The female louse lays six to eight eggs a day, which take ten days to hatch, so it isn't! Even if you get the louse, you won't get the eggs. Continue to fine comb the hair – for up to twenty minutes – every two days, for two to three weeks, to be sure the infection has cleared. Remember, it only takes one or two stray eggs hatching, for the infection to start again. That is why it is so hard to treat. As a good preventive rule, you should think about combing your hair once every month in this way and getting your family members to do the same.

TEA TREE OIL: Using a tea tree oil shampoo regularly should cleanse the scalp, soothe any irritation (because lice have fed on the scalp it can become infected) and generally help keep the scalp free of lice.

TURMERIC: Turmeric does have a history of killing lice, when it is made into a paste with Neem. But you would have to ask at your health shop to see if they have any shampoos containing this herb.

INTERESTING FACTS: The diarist Samuel Pepys certainly knew about lice, as did most sixteenth- and seventeenth-century writers. Robert Burns was obviously so taken with them he wrote a whole poem to one. In the seventeenth century there were 'lice houses' where you could go and spend the afternoon having them removed. It would have been far simpler to cut your hair, you might think – well, yes, but as often as not it was the wig that was being treated!

Lower back pain

The bane, or should I say pain, of many people's lives, lower back pain is one of these awful things that can strike anyone, anytime. I won't say anywhere. If you're reading this, then you'll know where. You'll also know that no one seems to know exactly what causes it in some cases, still less what to do about it. I suffered myself, many years ago, and the cause of it was a complete mystery, I have to say, to everyone including myself. I also have clients who are at their wits end, because they've been in agony for months. This is what I generally recommend.

PREVENTION: Obviously, if you're going to generally kill yourself by lugging great heavy weights about all morning, dig for hours in the garden in the afternoon, and shift whole rooms about before supper, then you're going to have a sore back by bedtime. Seriously, many sore backs are caused by strain. Always lift heavy items properly by crouching down and pushing up rather than bending over and slipping a disc. If you have a job that involves sitting for hours in one rather cramped position, make sure you sit straight, don't slouch then hope to look like anything other than a hunchbacked crab when you stand up. Also, try and get up regularly and move around. In saying all this, however, I must add that often people who suffer pain do none of these things.

CALCIUM: Make sure you get plenty of this if you suffer from a sore back. Eat lots of green leafy vegetables, basil, and thyme or take supplements to ensure that the bones are staying healthy.

PINEAPPLE: This fruit is very good for helping reduce inflammation. Indeed, many athletes swear by it to help them stay fit and get over injuries. So eating it regularly could help a little. The magic ingredient is bromelain, which can also be bought from health shops.

GINGER: Ginger also contains anti-inflammatory properties and is useful for treating arthritis, so might be helpful here. Try taking it as a capsule as well as adding it to your food. (See Ginger, page 175.)

A WORD OF CAUTION: Please refer to the individual remedy for further information to see if it is suitable for you.

INTERESTING FACT: Traditionally oats, cooked with vinegar and applied to the affected area, were used to treat back pain.

Menopause

'To be or not to be? That is the question.' Whether to suffer the sweats and flushes, mood swings and depression: to be on HRT or not. Well, it's the big one for our times, if you're a woman going through 'that time of life'. That's as opposed to 'having the time of your life'. Because for most women the menopause isn't 'the time of their lives'. It's when the hormones kick off, so to speak, and the hot flushes start, together with the night sweats, irritability, insomnia, headaches and dry skin. Of course, some women are very lucky and some just soldier on. The most commonly shared aspects of it are usually the flushes and sweats. Until you've experienced them you don't think they're possible. They're just something to giggle about when you're young and you hear middle-aged women complaining about 'the dreaded change'. Then you get older and you start to dread experiencing 'the change' yourself. Then you wake up night after night, drenched. In the morning you shower and ten minutes later you have another flush. It's impossible to feel fresh. As for the other discomforts – well, what do you do? It's not as if we can talk about 'prevention' as such here! Once you've reached a certain age the menopause *will* start. First of all, let's look at diet.

DIET: Believe it or not, in certain cultures, menopausal symptoms are unknown. Vegetarian cultures in particular, though that's not to say you should rush off and become a vegetarian if it's not for you. You could, however, consider eating plenty of black beans, soy beans and bean sprouts. They're high on things that help prevent flushes and strengthen the bone, which is another worry about reaching the menopause. Other foods to eat that contain substances that can help the body circulate oestrogen are strawberries, peaches, cabbages, tomatoes, apples, pears, broccoli, celery, parsley and fennel.

BLACK COHOSH: This is one I recommend for hot flushes and night sweats. It's actually approved in Germany for just this and studies have shown it's as effective as conventional drugs. If you don't fancy HRT and are suffering, then try this. The usual dosage is one tablet 500–600 mg, three times a day. (See Black cohosh, page 135.)

LICORICE: Most licorice sweets you see don't contain licorice, so ask at your health shop. Long-term use of too much licorice can cause problems, but there are safe daily doses. (See Licorice, page 195.)

CHINESE ANGELICA: Also known as Dang-quai, this has an age-old reputation for helping relieve hot flushes, vaginal dryness and irritation. Ask at your health shop.

A WORD OF CAUTION: Please refer to the remedy you choose for any cautions.

INTERESTING FACT: Black cohosh was used by native Americans for women's complaints for hundreds of years.

Menstrual cramps

Menstrual cramps are one of the major problems of the menstrual cycle. Really severe ones can floor the sufferer because they can be accompanied by nausea, very heavy bleeding and vomiting. Fibroids, especially in women over the age of 35, can be a cause of both cramps and excessive bleeding and I would advise anyone who thinks they might have them to have this checked immediately. The kind of problem I'm looking at here is the more simple misery that afflicts women, often even quite young women who have just started their periods, and the herbal remedies that are available for it.

PREVENTION: This is very difficult. Sometimes you can be fine one month and terrible the next. In some instances stress or trauma can make things worse, as can over working or being on your feet a lot. Then there's diet. Some herbalists and nutritionists put cramps down to a lack of certain minerals. Whatever, you should find the following remedies helpful.

RASPBERRY: Raspberry leaf tea is well known for helping ease cramps. It's a muscle relaxant and therefore helps to calm things down. The thing to do is keep a box handy and drink two or three cups a day just before your period is due to start, and also for the first day or so after it has started.

STRAWBERRY: Strawberry leaf tea has much the same effect. You'll note I'm saying the leaf here, rather than the berry. That's because it contains lots of vitamins. If you can't find the tea then boil some strawberry leaves in water, strain, allow to cool, and drink.

EVENING PRIMROSE OIL: This is good for most menstrual problems. While it might not always stop cramps, it does much to regulate the flow if taken according to the instructions. This is helpful because many menstrual cramps are due to heavy bleeding. (See Evening primrose oil, page 165.)

GINGER: This remarkable herb contains six pain-relieving compounds, so it's well worth trying. Look for a tea or tablets and take just before and during the first few days of your period. (See Ginger, page 175.)

BILBERRY: Either look for an extract or try eating a bowl of fresh bilberries. Apart from being very good for you, bilberry contains chemicals that relax muscles. (See Bilberry, page 134.)

KAVA KAVA: Because this herb contains two pain-relieving chemicals as well as other relaxant ones, it's also worth a try.

A WORD OF CAUTION: Always refer to the individual remedy you choose for information on any cautions and don't take any food type remedy if you're allergic to it.

INTERESTING FACT: It seems every culture has its own ideas on this one. The Chinese recommend Dang-quai (Chinese Angelica) for cramps. The Native American Indians use Squaw Vine. In the UK there are still many people who swear by a hot water bottle and a glass of sherry!

Migraine

A migraine is much more than a sore head. It is a crippling, often blinding, headache accompanied by nausea, vomiting and visual disturbance. In some cases no pain may be present, just an inability to see properly. Everything is fringed in black zigzags, like a cartoon drawing. Scarily, half the sight of the eye is missing. You look but you don't see. In others, the pain is so severe the sufferer can be hospitalised and doctors are stumped. One of the problems is that everyone is different. What triggers it in one sufferer might not affect another. What helps with one does absolutely nothing for someone else. Different things cause it too, which make it harder to find a definite, overall 'cure'. Let's just assume there are none as such. Bad news, I know. But not for everyone. I would say these headaches fall into categories and that it is possible to help some of them. I know. I've had a few myself. I've also seen the misery they cause.

PREVENTION: It's a fact that some migraines are triggered by an allergy to certain foods. If you are a sufferer, then look at your diet first of all. Do the attacks start after eating a particular food? If they do, then cut out that food. Sometimes, for whatever reason, your body can't break down the substances that are present and the migraine may be the result.

HORMONES: There is little known reason as to why many pregnant women, pre-menstrual women and young women (i.e. those starting their periods for the first time) are prone to migraines. So are women on the pill. This would suggest some kind of hormonal imbalance. If you fall into this category, then keep reading! There are things you can do.

DIET: Adding thyme, turmeric, garlic and ginger generally, can help fight a headache.

FEVERFEW: Feverfew is one of those herbs that can help migraine. (See Feverfew, page 169.)

EVENING PRIMROSE OIL: Long associated with menstrual problems, if you are a woman and your migraine is hormonal associated (i.e. it occurs as above), then taking extracts might help. (See Evening primrose oil, page 165.)

GINGKO BILOBA: In some instances, a migraine is triggered by abnormal blood flow. Because it improves blood flow generally, you could certainly try taking extracts on a regular basis. (See Gingko biloba, page 177.)

MAGNESIUM: I find it interesting that magnesium can also improve pre-menstrual tension. If you suffer from migraines you may have a magnesium deficiency. Magnesium generally helps relax cramps and spasms, so may help doubly here. (See Magnesium, page 198.)

SUGAR: Now I know this sounds strange, but a friend of mine came home from holiday one year with a beauty of a migraine. The most probable cause was dehydration – an overnight, nine-hour flight, no sleep, time difference, etc. Out of sheer desperation and because she couldn't see out of one eye, she took a teaspoon of sugar, and *voilà*! Within ten minutes the headache had gone. If your migraine is caused by tiredness, stress, or something like this, try doing the same, unless you're diabetic of course. If you can, sprinkle the sugar with ginger, as this will also alleviate the nausea.

A WORD OF CAUTION: Please remember to take any supplements according to instruction, particularly if you are pregnant. Remember, unless it is caused by low blood sugar levels, there is no good trying to help a migraine once it has struck. If you suffer and are trying the above, you must use herbal remedies regularly. Remember, too, a migraine can be caused by many different things. If the cause can be isolated, then the above may be helpful. Also, make sure you are treating a migraine. If you experience any sudden violent headache of the kind you have never had before, see a doctor.

INTERESTING FACT: Three times as many women experience migraines as men.

Morning sickness

Okay you're pregnant and hopefully everything is wonderful, then you get up in the morning and you feel sick. You go to work and you feel sick. You come home and you feel sick. You go to bed and you feel sick. You don't understand why it's called morning sickness when it lasts all day. You get up next morning and it's the same. A misery? You're right, it's a misery. Nobody told you how bad this is and though things do tend to settle after the first three months, you might be one of the unlucky few who proceed to experience morning sickness right to the time the baby is born. Can you do anything? Well hopefully yes, there are some remedies that might ease things for you. I hope they do. Having spent one of my pregnancies with my head hanging out the car window and in any convenient basin I could find, the whole time, you can certainly say I understand and sympathise. Lots!

DIET: Diet can help. Eat small meals rather than large, and eat frequently. Dry toast or crackers are good when you get up. If something is definitely disagreeing with you, even if it's your favourite food, then stop eating it. Don't ask me why, but even certain colours made me ill. That meant an entire repaint job on half the house!

GINGER: Ginger is wonderful for stopping nausea generally, be that motion sickness or just plain nausea. You could certainly try it and if it works, great. It can be taken as a tea – ask at your health shop – or add a small sprinkling to your own tea. It can also be taken on food. There's a carrots and ginger recipe in the recipe section, to give you the idea. If you don't like carrots, you can amend this to the vegetable of your choice. A glass of ginger ale, too, might help settle things down.

CABBAGE: Again, this is a traditional remedy for a stomach upset. Either raw or cooked, try adding it to your diet on a regular basis. A helping of coleslaw with your meals, for example, may improve things for you.

RASPBERRY: Raspberry is good for many women's 'troubles'. If I had known this when I had my terrible pregnancy, I'd have taken a cup of raspberry tea every day, perhaps with a sprinkling of ginger in it. The leaves contain a constituent that relaxes the uterus muscles.

PEPPERMINT: Sucking a peppermint stick might help. Again, this is one that generally relieves an upset stomach, so you could find, if your sickness isn't too severe, that you feel better.

CITRUS FRUITS: Try putting a piece of orange rind in your tea. It's old wife stuff I know, but some reports indicate it does help.

A WORD OF CAUTION: Don't drink large amounts of peppermint tea if you are pregnant. In some instances this has triggered a miscarriage. Also, don't go daft with the ginger for the same reason. One gram is all you need for morning sickness purposes. You'd have to take an awful lot to bring on a miscarriage but often when you're ill you're desperate. Otherwise, the above are all safe to take. Obviously, if you experience violent vomiting over a short period of time you must consult your doctor.

INTERESTING FACT: We all have a great many theories about why women suffer morning sickness. However, there has never been any scientific fact as to the true cause.

Motion sickness

If you've ever experienced this then you'll know what a misery it is. For years, every holiday I took seemed to involve a particular member of my family being very sick to the extent that a four-hour journey could take ten, and I have memories of stopping at every lay-by and field we passed, to haul fresh clothes from the suitcases and mop the car. Some people just have it on a particular form of transport, or if that form of transport is having a bumpy ride. Others just travel badly, a great worry to their travelling companions when a journey has to be undertaken. The symptoms are obviously vomiting, as the name suggests, but they don't just stop there. Sometimes the vomiting is so severe and prolonged, dizziness and general queasiness join in, and you begin to wish you were anywhere rather than here. In fact, you even start wishing you were dead! You can't help thinking it's the most expensive chuck up in history, when you consider the costs involved and sometimes the back yard has never looked more welcoming!

PREVENTION: Well, as with some other ailments here, there's a very obvious prevention. Just don't travel! But that's a lot easier said than done. We all spend our lives hopping in and out of cars, trains, boats and planes and sometimes, for no apparent reason, we can suddenly experience a bout of motion sickness on transport we've used with no side effects ever before. Generally, there's not a lot you can do to prevent it, but some things can be done to stop it getting worse. For example, if you're a regular sufferer, then don't eat heavy meals before you take your journey. Snack on light foods and drink water. Fizzy drinks and alcohol are murder to digest if you're a poor traveller. Alcohol dehydrates, especially in planes. If you're on a train, sit facing the way you are travelling. Sometimes it helps actually to look out the window and see the way you are going. Reading isn't a good idea if you suffer motion sickness, especially in a car. Letting plenty of air circulate on a car journey helps. Also, if you have a child who suffers – and many more children than adults tend to suffer motion sickness when in cars – don't race. Wheeling round bends, bouncing over bumps and racing to overtake the car in front isn't going to help junior keep the contents of their stomach under control, now is it? Also, make frequent stops just to take in fresh air and let them walk about. Motion sickness is so terribly distressing that many people get a 'thing' about travelling, and knowing before they set out that you're only going to drive half an hour then stop for five minutes, can help them overcome this, because they feel a sense of achievement in managing that half hour. Remember, too, be prepared. That's not just a brownie motto. It's always a good idea to have plenty of wipes, tissues, towels, etc. with you.

GINGER: Ginger is very good for motion sickness and many motion sickness tablets contain it. You can try asking at your health shop for ginger capsules and take them according to the instructions before your journey (if you wait till you're actually sick, they won't do much good). Alternatively, you can take half a teaspoon of ginger. Ginger also comes as a tea. A cup before you go might just be the thing. (See Ginger, page 175.)

PEPPERMINT: This is good for stopping retching, so a cup of peppermint tea before you travel might help the stomach muscles relax. (See Peppermint, page 215.)

CINNAMON: Cinnamon also prevents nausea, so adding a sprinkling to your tea could do the trick. (See Cinnamon, page 152.)

A WORD OF CAUTION: Avoid peppermint or cinnamon if you're pregnant.

INTERESTING FACT: The word nausea comes form the Greek word for ship. I think I can see why!

Mouth ulcers

Traditionally, mouth ulcers were said to be a sign of telling lies. A sort of early version of the Pinocchio story and not much consolation for any poor sufferer, I'm sure! They can actually be very annoying and painful too, particularly when on the tongue. If you're a sufferer you'll know well what I'm talking about here – small white spots on the inside of the cheek, tongue or lip. You'll also know that, as in all good horror stories, sometimes they come back.

PREVENTION: Some ulcers are caused by eating spicy food. So if you're a regular sufferer and fond of hot curries, then there's your answer, I'm afraid. Another reason is stress. Generally that can lead to all kinds of things going wrong with the body because it has to find a way of dealing with tension. Some people, too, have a habit of biting their lips and the inside of their cheeks. Then they're very surprised when an ulcer develops! For those guilty parties, and I'm sure you know who you are, there are some things you can do!

ALOE VERA: A dab of Aloe Vera gel on the affected area can help to reduce the pain. (See Aloe Vera, page 121.)

GOLDENSEAL: This herb was traditionally used by the American Indians to treat wounds. The name alone suggests that it was sure to be good for mending sores, so I wouldn't hesitate to recommend it for healing troublesome mouth ulcers. Either ask for an ointment containing it at your health shop, or buy the dried herb, put a teaspoonful in a cup of boiling water, allow to cool, and rinse the mouth. You could try this three times a day. The special antiseptic qualities in goldenseal should soon do the trick.

MAGNESIUM: If you suffer regularly from mouth ulcers, then magnesium supplements could help. It may even be that you are deficient in some way and this is why you have them so often. (See Magnesium, page 198.)

SAGE: A strong cup of sage tea can cure both mouth and throat if it is also ulcerated. Put one teaspoon of the dried herb in a cup of boiling water, allow to cool, strain, and then use to rinse the mouth. Alternatively, you can try boiling a teaspoonful of dried sage in 1 litre of water, allow to cool, strain and add two drops of tincture of myrrh. Rub the affected area with the mixture. (See Sage, page 227.)

A WORD OF CAUTION: Please remember to refer to the individual remedy to make sure it is the right one for you.

INTERESTING FACT: In 'the old days' salt was used to cure mouth ulcers.

Prostate enlargement

The prostate gland is most definitely a 'male thing'. One that when men are young doesn't seem to cause too many problems. Unfortunately, like certain other parts of the male anatomy, it can't stop growing! That's where the problems start – often round about the age of 50. As it grows it starts to pinch the urethra, causing difficulty in emptying the bladder properly. If you have to get up several times a night to urinate, then the chances are you've got this problem. It's one of the main symptoms. Another is getting any kind of forceful flow.

PREVENTION: Obviously you can't stop a gland from growing, so sadly there isn't really anything I can suggest here. Because of the nature of this problem, many men are shy of seeking help. Don't be. It's much worse to struggle on with something you're worried about, that is spoiling your life in some ways, than make an appointment to check out that this is what's wrong with you. Prostate cancer often claims lives unnecessarily because men have neglected a prostate condition, or been too embarrassed to seek advice. I'm looking at the non-cancerous enlargement here and hope I'm not setting any alarm bells ringing. Once you've had the condition checked out, and know this is all it is, there are drugs the doctor can prescribe. But maybe you'd like to try some herbal remedies too.

NETTLE: Some studies actually show that nettle extracts taken from the root help prevent the conversion of too much testosterone in the body, thus improving the condition significantly. This is if the extracts are taken daily. Please ask at your health shop for nettle root extract and take according to the instructions. (See Nettle, page 207.)

LICORICE: Licorice is also good for keeping the testosterone levels down. The only problem is that, in some instances, people take too much and taking too much can lead to headaches, lethargy and water retention. The best thing I would say, is to ask at your health shop for extracts containing it and take according to the instructions. You would have to take a lot over a long period of time to experience a problem. Obviously, if you are taking it and you start having these symptoms, you should stop. (See Licorice, page 195.)

ZINC: There are some studies to suggest that zinc can reduce the size of the prostate. It comes in tablet form as a supplement and might certainly be worth trying. If you're going to use it, you can try discussing it with your doctor first, to see if you're a mild to moderate case, because that's where it's most helpful. Supplements are available from health shops and supermarkets. Please follow the guidelines. Taking too much can lead to nausea and vomiting. A dose of 30 mg a day is generally sufficient. (See Zinc, page 255.)

A WORD OF CAUTION: Please refer to the individual remedy for appropriate advice on dosage.

INTERESTING FACT: Pumpkin seeds are used in Turkey and the Ukraine. Interestingly they contain zinc.

Scrapes

Sorry, we've no remedy here for those of you who are always getting into one! We're talking skin scrapes here! You'll know exactly what these look like and how they happen and the good news is you can't honestly prevent them, unless you sit on a chair all day and don't move! There are, however, a few things you can do if you've got one. First of all it's important to give it a gentle sponge over with water, to remove any grit or dirt that may have got trapped in it. Then you should think about a cream. Whether you cover it up is up to you. I always think it's a good idea to keep things covered for a day or so, to let them heal and keep any infection or germs from getting in. But I know everyone is different.

CALENDULA: Creams containing calendula are obtainable from health shops and you will find that calendula is very good at healing wounds. You can even throw some petals in boiling water, steep, allow to cool, and wash the scrape with it. (See Calendula, page 144.)

ECHINACEA: Echinacea can be applied to the skin. It contains antiseptic qualities as well as helping to boost the immune system. If you have a tincture, dab a little on a cloth and put it on the scrape. (See Echinacea, page 161.)

TEA TREE OIL: Tea tree oil can certainly help heal and clean a cut or scrape. The only problem is that sometimes it can sting – as many non-herbal antiseptics do! If you do use it, just be ready for that. (See Tea tree oil, page 233.)

COMFREY: While I would never recommend the taking of comfrey, you can certainly rub some fresh leaves on a scrape or look for a cream containing it. It has many healing qualities. (See Comfrey, page 154.)

A WORD OF CAUTION: Never take tea tree oil or comfrey. One is highly toxic, the other can cause liver damage. They are for external use only. Also, if you have hayfever you may be allergic to calendula. If you develop a rash, then stop using the treatment.

INTERESTING FACT: Iodine was widely used in the first half of the last century to treat scrapes. And my own recent research has proved, to me at least, that this mineral is invaluable, if a little difficult to obtain.

Sea-sickness (see motion sickness)

Shingles

Shingles is the ghost of chickenpox past and like all good ghosts is much scarier than the original thing. While the blisters heal after a week or so, the pain goes on for months, years sometimes, and can be severe – this is called postherpetic neuralgia for those of you who are unlucky enough to get it. I'm going to cover this as well in this section and also look at some things that keep the immune system healthy. It's a well-known fact that while no one knows exactly what triggers the shingles virus it is most common amongst people with poor immune systems.

PREVENTION: Shingles derives from chickenpox. What happens is that after getting chickenpox the virus remains in the nerve cells of the body, flaring years later, for reasons that remain a mystery to some extent. In some instances people report developing shingles after coming into contact with someone with chickenpox, so if you're elderly, and one of your grandchildren has chickenpox, it might be an idea to stay away. Other people just develop it anyway. If you take things like gingko biloba and ginseng, herbals that boost the immune system, then you are lessening your chances of getting shingles, as it tends to flare when the immune system is weak. If you do develop shingles, your first port of call is your doctor, who will then prescribe a course of treatment. Below are some herbals you can try too. Dietwise, food for the invalid should include plenty of pears. Pear juice is full of antiviral acid – just the thing to help you get on your feet. Other foods that might help are soy beans, lentils, spinach, peas, fenugreek and parsley.

LICORICE: Licorice is good for shingles sufferers. But I'm not meaning the sweet candy, which can be bought here. Look for a tea, ointment or supplement. The ointment, which can be hard to come by, is good for healing the blisters. If you can't get it, you can dab the tea on instead, in addition to drinking it. (See Licorice, page 195.)

RED PEPPER (CAYENNE POWDER): This is one for postherpetic neuralgia and, rather than looking for a cream containing Capsaicin which is the painkiller that red pepper contains, just mix some powdered red pepper (cayenne powder) with any white skin lotion until it turns pink, then dab it on.

LEMON BALM: Some herbalists recommend this for herpes, which is a very similar virus to the one that causes shingles, so I'd say it's worth a try. Either look for a tea containing it and, as with licorice, drink it or dab it on the blisters. Alternatively, you can make your own by steeping a teaspoon of dried extract in a cup of water and applying it to the sores.

VALERIAN: This is a mild sedative and ideal for helping you relax and get off to sleep to escape the irritation. (See Valerian, page 239.)

A WORD OF CAUTION: Please refer to the individual remedy. Licorice in particular is a very powerful herbal and must be used according to instruction.

INTERESTING FACT: The Chinese use Chinese Angelica or Dang-quai to treat shingles, although traditionally this herb was used for menstrual problems.

Sinusitis

Sinusitis is inflammation of the cavities surrounding the nasal passages – one that causes severe pain across the nose and cheeks, and sometimes a headache too. Usually it develops after a cold, or flu, but it can come about after hayfever or a dental infection. However it is caused, it can be difficult to get rid of.

PREVENTION: This is really not possible unless you manage not to catch a cold – although you could try some of the herbal remedies mentioned below, if you do have a cold. You never know, they just might stop sinusitis developing.

EUCALYPTUS: You can try adding a few drops of essential eucalyptus oil to a hot bath and steeping yourself in it. It's certainly a nice relaxing way to clear those sinuses!

OLBAS OIL: Olbas oil is something of an 'in thing' at the moment and very useful, too, for treating this kind of infection according to many of my clients who have found relief by using it. Simply inhale according to the instructions.

MINT: Any of the mints are helpful in clearing up this condition – oregano, mint and peppermint in particular. All of them contain antiseptic qualities. Just try making a cup of peppermint tea and inhaling the vapours as you drink it. Or, if you have the essential oils, you could burn them. Just remember not to make your cup of tea with the oils. They are for external use only.

ECHINACEA: This herb is excellent for boosting the immune system and clearing up all kinds of infections. What's more, it's so easily come by. It's well worth a try if you suffer from sinusitis or have a cold and want it to clear. (See Echinacea, page 161.)

GOLDENSEAL: Goldenseal capsules are very good for treating infections, being a sort of herbal antibiotic, so you should find them helpful here.

A WORD OF CAUTION: Remember to refer to the individual instructions for each remedy and follow them.

INTERESTING FACT: Some herbalists suggest taking a spoonful of horseradish to cure sinusitis. I think you'd have to be pretty brave! It sounds like more kill than cure to me, but you could try it on your food.

Stings

Stings are something else I associate with summer and holidays. Probably because the first time I ever got stung I was on a remote island and ended up with a leg like a balloon – all within minutes. I was frightened, I can tell you! It was one of these times when getting away from it all didn't seem such a good idea and I just wished I'd holed up in some hotel with the rest of Europe! If only I'd known about herbal medicine in these days! But I do now and here's what I'd do.

PREVENTION: Of course this sounds silly. You can't always prevent a dirty great wasp from stinging you, if that is its intention. You can, however, wear a repellent if you're abroad. I always do because the mosquitoes also love me. Insects don't like citrus smells, so anything containing lemon is good to use. Basil leaves rubbed on the skin also keep insects away. So does tea tree oil dabbed on the skin. But it has to be the oil.

IF YOU'RE STUNG: Some people are allergic to certain insect stings. The problem, as I found out, is that you don't know this till you're stung. Certainly you'll know once you're stung. If the area starts to swell horrendously, then you have an allergy and it may be you would have to carry anti-histamine tablets with you as a matter of course. Extract the sting, if it is present, by squeezing the part firmly, or use a pair of tweezers. Apply an ice-pack to stop the swelling. If the area becomes red then it is infected and you would need to apply an antiseptic cream. There are herbal ones. (See Antiseptic, page 125.)

CALENDULA: The flowers of this plant can help to reduce the pain.

Simply rub them on the skin or keep a cream containing calendula in your medicine cupboard. (See Calendula, page 144.)

ONION: Applying chopped onion to a sting can help to relieve the pain and swelling. Obviously, if someone has been stung, you don't have time to stand and boil the skins. But it's something you could do later to relieve the pain. (See Onion, page 210.)

CAMOMILE: Camomile can help to reduce inflammation. (See Camomile, page 145.) Try soaking a tea bag and applying it to the infected area.

A WORD OF CAUTION: Please refer to the individual pages for the remedies listed above. If you are stung in the throat area you should see a doctor. If it swells it could cause problems breathing. Also, if you experience any violent reaction to being stung, don't mess about trying to put on calendula flowers and boil onions, get yourself to a doctor immediately.

Stress

What makes writing this book so interesting is that when you take a look at some of the ailments that were top of the list with other generations, stress isn't one of them. Of course that doesn't mean it didn't exist previously. In some shape or form it's probably always existed, but never so much as now. And that's largely down to the way people live. Hectic in the extreme, shall we say? So, if you're reading this section, it stands to reason you know what stress is and you think you've got it. At its best, stress can be something we joke about when we go on a shopping trip and can't find a parking space – just a short-term feeling. At its worst it can make us irritable, bad tempered with everyone, nervous, unable to sleep, unable to think, panicky and really just plain awful! Moreover, although a certain amount of stress does no harm, and in some rather strange ways can be good, feeling that way in the long-term is damaging. So let's look at some of the things that might help.

PREVENTION: Some people just have 'stressful' personalities and that is very difficult to change. For example, you might be the kind of person who worries about everything and anything. Even a simple thing, like cancelling a visit to a friend, can stress you out, largely because you can't decide what to do about it, or are concerned about causing offence. So, obviously, if you do get hugely stressed by bigger things, it's going to be very difficult for you. If this is you, then perhaps you would benefit from some kind of therapy or counselling. Meditation could be useful, for example, helping you control these impulses, as could yoga or any of those therapies that involve relaxation. Even just a few sessions could be sufficient to set you on the way to the 'new you', so to speak, and could help you to learn ways to control your breathing and relax more when you start to feel you can't cope with things, or face things.

Moving on from the 'stressful' personality, some people just go through times when they are stressed. This could be down to their work – certain professions have high 'casualties' in this regard, taking many prisoners – and again it might be that there is nothing you can do about this, in which case you need to learn other ways of managing how you feel. One of the most important things to do if you have a difficult job is to find other things to do that take you completely away from it. This could be anything, from learning a musical instrument to joining a club. That way you have something else to think about other than work. Hopefully it becomes something to look forward to and a goal you can set yourself. It's very important to switch off in life, otherwise we're not doing ourselves any good. So bear this in mind.

Other forms of stress can be created by certain situations. The death of a loved one, moving house, or divorce are all fairly high on the list here. And it's important to recognise that often we are falling to pieces with good cause, that certain things are beyond our control, and to try things to help keep us calm in the meantime, because hopefully that time will pass. If, for whatever reason, you are suffering stress, then there are a few herbal remedies you can take that should help things considerably and also have the advantage of being non-addictive.

BACH'S RESCUE REMEDY: Dr Bach's Flower Remedies are good for all kinds of things and yes, stress is one of them. They are also very easy to come by at your health shop. Just look for the one for stress and take accordingly to instructions. (See Bach Flower Remedies, page 130.)

ST JOHN'S WORT: St John's Wort has the reputation of being a sort of herbal happy pill. It's compounds help cheer you up generally but they also help you relax.

CAMOMILE: A cup of camomile tea taken once or twice a day can calm you down if you're feeling stressed. It also helps you sleep better at night if you find you can't, thus helping you function better during the day. (See Camomile, page 145.)

VALERIAN: Like camomile, valerian is a non-addictive relaxant. If you take it at bedtime, it should help you get to sleep without knocking you out. It should also ensure you sleep better. Varelian can be taken during the day too. Just put six or seven drops in water. (See Valerian, page 239.)

LAVENDER: This is a good relaxant. You can try putting a handful in a bath, burning the oil, or sleeping on a lavender-filled pillow. (See Lavender, page 192.)

A WORD OF CAUTION: Please refer to the remedy you choose for any cautions.

INTERESTING FACT: Stress is now a major cause of absenteeism in the workplace.

Sunburn

Well, we all know how it is. It's a lovely day outside and we just can't resist it. Out we go, and of course we've bunged the sun cream on. But it's just so nice. And the skin's not the least bit red. What's another hour? And another one? And maybe one after that? The skin's still fine. Everything is wonderful. Then the sun goes away. We come indoors. 'Oh dear! Who's that funny creature in the mirror?' we think. 'Is it a lobster? Is it a crab?' The bad news is it's us, and worse is to come! As burns go most sunburns aren't too bad, although some can be terrible. How do I know? Well, I once burned my legs, sitting by the pool on holiday one year. I couldn't walk for hours. The skin on my legs actually felt as if it was shrinking. Being in the sun means being sensible, otherwise you can make yourself very unwell, in addition to increasing the risk of skin cancer. Nobody's saying don't do it. Being in the sun is also good for the health. But there are some things you should do first.

PREVENTION: Prevention is very definitely better than cure for this one. Always use a sun cream and pay attention to what it says on the bottle about how long you can stay in the sun wearing it. If you are going to be in the water, check to see if your cream is water resistant and apply it frequently if it's not. There is less shade if you are out in a boat or canoe, and that's when many people do get burned. The rays are most damaging between eleven and two. That's when all the sensible people who live in hot countries stay indoors. That's also when I notice all the British holidaymakers out in force, frying their bodies as if there was no tomorrow. Well, for some there won't be. Sorry to sound like the party-pooper here, but skin cancer is very much on the increase. You can still stay in the sun. but stay under the parasol, or put on a light top. Remember, too, you never actually feel yourself getting burned. It's hours later when you notice and it's too late to stop it then. Also, drink lots of water or juice, or you're going to suffer more than sunburn. Alcohol dehydrates. Wear a hat. And never, never fall asleep. On holiday one year there was a case of a man who did just that and spent the rest of the week in hospital with third-degree burns.

ALOE VERA: Okay, so despite everything you've got a burn. The skin is nipping, hot and red. This soothing green gel is very good at cooling the skin and helping it to heal. I always keep a bottle in the cupboard and pack it in my holiday luggage every year. Try to do the same. (See Aloe Vera, page 121.)

CALENDULA: Calendula flowers speed the healing of wounds. Look in your health shop for a cream containing it. (See Calendula, page 144.)

WITCH HAZEL: I'm very fond of witch hazel as a healing ointment. It's another one I keep in the medicine cupboard. You can try applying it on a cloth to the burned area. (See Witch hazel, page 252.)

CUCUMBER: If you've nothing else immediately to hand but do have this, then simply slice it open and apply it.

VITAMIN E: This does help with burned skin. Look for a cream containing it.

A WORD OF CAUTION: Please refer to the individual pages for your chosen remedy, as there are things you should be aware of with each.

INTERESTING FACT: The Chinese recommend both sipping green tea and applying it to the burn to help sunburn.

Tendinitis

Tendinitis is an inflammation of the tendons, the tissues that connect the muscles to the bones, something we all tend to have a bit of a giggle about because of the funny names it's known by – Tennis Elbow being one. That's until we've got it ourselves, that is. Then we see how very painful it is and also how difficult it is to get rid of. Nor does it necessarily have anything to do with playing tennis. I've had it and I've never lifted a racket in my life! Well, not quite! For hundreds of years this kind of joint pain was endured by people who worked hard on the land and at home. They probably knew the herbal remedies better than anyone. And it's some of these I'm therefore going to list. Ice-packs can also help reduce the swelling till some of the remedies get going.

PREVENTION: This is very difficult because a lot of tendinitis is caused by using the joint repetitively, and also by people who do genuinely play a lot of sports with arm movements. I was only kidding about the tennis!

ECHINACEA: Some herbalists recommend taking a few drops of echinacea tincture daily until the swelling and pain have gone. (See Echinacea, page 161.)

COMFREY: Because it contains anti-inflammatory compounds comfrey can be used to treat tendinitis. However, a tea would work better than a cream, because you can soak the affected joint in it. But this is one tea I wouldn't recommend you drink (see Comfrey, page 154). If you can get some comfrey leaves, however, let them sit in a bowl of hot water then bathe the sore area.

LICORICE: Here's a sweet one, so to speak. Licorice does contain anti-inflammatory compounds, so if you've got tendinitis you might like to pay a visit to your health shop and see what extract is for you. Licorice tea can be quite effective and it is generally safe to take two or three times a day. (See Licorice, page 195.)

SAGE: Generally, bathing in a sage bath can reduce aches and pains and is especially good for sport's injuries and tiredness. You can also try adding eight drops of essential sage oil to one tablespoon of sunflower oil and massaging into the affected joint. This should be repeated for several days. (See Sage, page 227.)

ROSEMARY: Rosemary oil can be used in exactly the same way as sage. (See above.)

PINEAPPLE: I'm sure all these athletes who eat pineapple regularly because they believe it helps reduce the problem of tendinitis must be onto something! Certainly it contains a substance that reduces inflammation, so it's worth giving it a try, although I would think you'd have to eat a lot of it to get the full benefit. If you do a lot of sports, however, it could be worth adding to your diet on a regular basis.

NETTLE: Nettle is so good for other painful conditions involving joints I would recommend it here. Ask at your health shop for a nettle tea to drink or bathe the joint in. Or make your own by adding nettle leaves to boiling water. Just remember to wear gloves when you go to pick the nettles! Once the nettle is boiled it soon loses its sting. (See Nettle, page 207.)

A WORD OF CAUTION: Please refer to theindividual remedy to be sure it is suitable for you and always take according to the instructions.

INTERESTING FACT: Traditionally, fresh cabbage leaves, whitened in boiling water, then wrapped round the injured limb were used to treat tendinitis. I don't know about treating it but the smell must have been terrible!

Thyroid

Right away I'm going to say that if you have a thyroid condition then your first step should be to the doctor and you must do whatever he or she says. Thyroid hormones regulate the metabolism of every cell in your body, so this isn't something to mess about with. The things I am going to recommend here won't solve it. They might help, but they must only be taken with your doctor's approval.

HYPERTHYROIDISM

This is when the thyroid is 'set on high' and there are high blood levels of thyroid hormones circulating the body. The symptoms are rapid pulse, profuse sweating, fatigue, bulging eyes, weight loss, irritability, muscle tremors and restlessness.

KELP: Hyperthyroidism is virtually unknown amongst the Japanese who eat a great deal of kelp with their food. Among those who have become Westernised, however, it is on the increase. Kelp might be worth a try therefore. It can be taken in tablet form or bought powdered and sprinkled on your food. (See Kelp, page 107.)

BROCCOLI: Broccoli contains substances that restrain the thyroid from producing too much hormone. So this is a good natural food you can try adding to your diet every day.

MELISSA: Studies show that Melissa (or lemon balm) can reduce thyroid hormone production – but this is by injection. You could, however, try taking it orally.

INTERESTING FACTS: Women tend to suffer much more than men. Hyperthyroidism is also called Graves' Disease, after the Irish physician who was first to identify it.

HYPOTHYROIDISM

Sounds just about the same as its partner, doesn't it? In this condition, however, the thyroid is 'set on low'. There are just not enough hormones circulating the body. The symptoms of this are different from the ones above. They include lethargy, depression, headaches and low body temperatures. So instead of springing around doing everything at a great pace you're much slower generally. You'll also suffer recurrent infections, find it difficult to lose weight and, if you're a woman, have painful periods.

KELP: Kelp can actually be useful for this condition, as it can for hyperthyroidism. It is high in iodine, which the body must have to produce thyroid hormones. Try sprinkling the dried powder on your food or taking tablets. Another food that contains iodine is mustard. Cabbage, soy beans, peanuts, oats and sesame seeds could also help.

WALNUT: This is a Turkish remedy and it's not quite as simple as just eating them or using walnut oil on your food, although you can certainly try that if you wish. What you need is the fresh juice of green walnuts and you get that by boiling them for 20 minutes, allowing the liquid to cool and drinking. Not very pleasant, I have to say.

ST JOHN'S WORT: This will not help your hypothyroidism. What it will do is help the depression and lethargy that accompanies it while you're waiting for the drugs you're on to take effect. If you're pregnant, however, you will need to find something else.

A WORD OF CAUTION: Please refer to the individual remedy you choose and please remember what I've said about seeing your doctor. In this instance, their advice is crucial and I am not recommending herbal medicine as an alternative but something that could help with whatever he or she suggests.

Tinnitus

Many people are familiar with tinnitus. It's the ringing or buzzing in your ears that you experience after coming into contact with loud or continuous noise. For most, the sensation doesn't last. When it goes on, however, it can be a nuisance. Experts are not altogether sure why it occurs but it is thought that it results from damage to the hair cells, which then affects the messages that go to the brain. This damage can result from a number of things. I'll look at some of these in a minute, but for some people tinnitus just strikes out of the blue, which is why it is such a mystery.

PREVENTION: Like many other ailments, it is possible to take simple precautions to avoid making things worse. If the ringing is being caused, for example, by coming into contact with noise, then try to avoid or limit going to noisy places as much as possible. This can be difficult. Even film soundtracks seem to be at the top of the decibel scale these days. On the whole, we are all living with so much more noise around us than previously. Just take a listen to the traffic if you don't believe me. Then there's the TV up full blare. The discos-on-wheels so many people drive along in. If you're at a noisy event one night, try to do something quiet the next. Keep the volume on personal stereos at a reasonable volume. If you're at a disco or party, stand away from the speakers. Don't be ashamed to wear earplugs if you're continually in a noisy environment. Rather suffer someone having a giggle, or having to keep saying 'Eh?', than develop this condition.

INGKO BILOBA: One theory about tinnitus is that it is caused by a deficiency of blood to the inner ear. In this case, gingko biloba taken once a day (120 mg) is thought to be helpful because it increases the blood flow. Indeed, one of my clients has tried this and found the tinnitus went away.

ZINC: Zinc deficiency also seems to be associated with tinnitus. While it can be difficult to take a lot of zinc, you can certainly try eating more foods that are good sources. These include spinach, cucumbers, parsley and asparagus. Or try our zinc soup. The recipe is on page 261.

INTERESTING FACT: The Chinese herbalists recommend sesame seeds sprinkled on foods for the treatment of tinnitus.

Ulcers

An ulcer is a sore. External ones can be dealt with by applying a little comfrey ointment or some of the other herbs mentioned in any of the skin 'condition' sections. There's also a section on mouth ulcers, if you're having trouble with those. What I want to look at here are stomach ulcers – a sore in the lining of the stomach, sometimes called a peptic ulcer. Peptic ulcers often bleed, causing sharp pain in the stomach or just below it. If you've got these symptoms, then it's important you see a doctor first, to check that this *is* an ulcer. You will almost certainly be given some kind of medicine to treat it. There are also some herbal remedies you can try and these are listed below. Changes to the diet can also help. Salt, for example, irritates the stomach, while sugar increases acidity. So both should perhaps be restricted if you want to do something about this condition. Other good foods are listed below.

PREVENTION: Various studies show that ulcers are caused by a bacterial infection but many people have these bacteria in their systems and it doesn't lead to ulcers. So why it triggers it in some is unclear. It is thought, however, that stress, alcohol abuse, smoking and poor diet may play a part – although, again, many people who don't smoke or drink develop peptic ulcers. Some ulcers have also been found to be a side effect of certain drugs. So really this is a difficult one and what I would say is to try to include certain foods in your diet – ones that have anti-ulcer properties. That way you should cut down on the risk of developing one. Diet can also play a part for those who have developed an ulcer.

DIET: Coffee, tea, alcohol and aspirin should be avoided if you have an ulcer. Very difficult I would say – all life's little pleasures gone! I wasn't meaning the aspirin of course, though it's very good for certain things. Ulcers, alas, aren't among them! Perhaps you could cut down your intake, along with sugar and salt, if you are a sufferer. Certain fruits, such as pineapple and banana, contain anti-ulcer properties, so, taken regularly, these could help prevent you developing a stomach ulcer. Garlic and red pepper, contrary to belief about what spices do to the stomach, are actually very good preventatives. All you need to do is sprinkle them onto your cooking. Bilberry helps the stomach produce a mucus that protects its lining. Teawise, camomile and green tea are the two I would recommend. Camomile contains substances that limit the growth of the bacteria that cause ulcers. Green tea is a digestive aid generally. However, licorice is also good as a preventative and what you could do is add a little of the dried herb to one of the others occasionally. Licorice root is also good for treating irritations of the stomach, so this might also be useful if you have actually developed an ulcer. (See Licorice, page 195.)

CABBAGE JUICE: Raw cabbage juice is an old folk remedy for ulcers – one that has been studied into the bargain! You would, however, have to drink quite a bit each day for up to two weeks. If you don't like it, as I suspect is more than likely to be the case, and are a bit worried about the intimate relationship you're probably going to strike up with your bathroom as a result, you can always try making cabbage soup instead!

RHUBARB: This is a Chinese remedy and therefore one I would trust. Rhubarb, however, is another of these foods that might cause you to become very intimately acquainted with your bathroom. Certainly constipation shouldn't be a problem. Seriously, if you find that after eating it you are developing diarrhoea, then cut back on the amount you are taking.

TURMERIC: Ask at your health shop for turmeric capsules. They're very good for relieving the burning sensation associated with ulcers.

MEADOWSWEET: This herbal aspirin is very good for treating ulcers. And yes, that's despite what I said a moment ago about aspirins. That's because Meadowsweet contains other properties, all of them ideal for treating this condition. It's also a very good digestive aid generally. (See Meadowsweet, page 201.)

A WORD OF CAUTION: Please refer to the individual remedy you choose to see if it's appropriate for you.

INTERESTING FACT: In India, banana powder has been used for hundreds of years to treat ulcers.

Warts

Well, now we come to something that most people have or have had at some time, or may well go on to get. Warts usually appear on the hands. Children especially, probably because of the amount of time they spend with each other, often have them. Warts come in various sizes, can be very unsightly, but seldom cause pain. That is unless you are unlucky enough to get them on the soles of your feet. They are a viral infection, which means that they are difficult to prevent. You can't, for example, have your child running about in gloves all the time! Sometimes, too, they're difficult to get rid of, short of having them 'burnt off' at a doctor's surgery. There are some remedies you can try, however, which might help.

DANDELION: Dandelion leaves and stems contain latex, which could help treat a small wart. Simply tear the leaves or stem and apply the white fluid that oozes out, to the affected area. Apply each day for up to ten days.

FIG: Historically, fig was used to teat boils, warts and corns. Squeeze the fig to extract the white fluid and apply to the wart. As with dandelion, you might need to do this several times to see a result.

PINEAPPLE: Pineapple is said to work in much the same way as fig.

Cut a square and tape to the affected area overnight. Then soak in hot water.

BASIL: Traditionally, basil was used to treat warts, but then so was just about everything else under the sun! If you have a basil plant in your garden, then try rubbing the leaves on the wart every day for a week.

THYME: The same goes for thyme. This is one I tried and found resulted in quite an improvement. Rub the leaves on the wart every day. Alternatively, tape some on with a sticking plaster.

A WORD OF CAUTION: Obviously if you've got a huge great wart that is bothering you, see a doctor. If any of the above cause itching or irritation to the skin, then stop using them. Otherwise they are perfectly safe to use as suggested.

INTERESTING FACT: Huckleberry Finn had his own ideas about curing warts in Mark Twain's book *The Adventures of Tom Sawyer*. He suggested a dead cat. I know no more!

Wrinkles

Isn't this something we all dread? Mainly, of course, it's all down to ageing, alas not something we can do all that much about, in some regards. Let's face it, the clock is always ticking! Wrinkles come about because of changes to the skin. As we get older the skin loses its elasticity, its ability to absorb moisture – something that keeps it looking young – and starts to line. Haven't you noticed, too, that it starts to line most on the bits that are most exposed? You don't see your feet looking like they're about one hundred now do you, or other well-covered parts? And that's the most annoying thing.

PREVENTION: Smokers and sun worshippers tend to line more quickly. I like the sun myself but I always put a lot of sun cream or moisturiser on my face and wear a hat, so hopefully I won't end up looking like a prune. If you have a particular habit of screwing your brow or knitting your eyebrows together, then you're going to develop wrinkles accordingly. A good healthy diet can help slow down the ageing process generally. Drinking lots of water keeps the skin nice and moist. Obviously, if you're going to stay up late and be 'out on the tiles', or indeed 'the randan', every night, then you're not going to look like a beautiful young thing in the morning. Maybe you might for a while – we can all pretend after all. But you can't indefinitely sustain that kind of lifestyle without it showing somewhere, and where it tends to show is your face. There are some herbal suggestions that are good for keeping the skin moistened, too. These are the ones I would suggest.

CUCUMBER: Yes, the patches on the eyes really work. It's not just people looking silly! Put one in your blender and apply as a face-mask for 30 minutes.

CARROT: This one's for eating. Generally, including carrots in your diet regularly gives you lots of vitamin A, which keeps skin moist. (See Carrot, page 147.)

OLIVE OIL: Olive oil has been used for thousands of years to soften the skin and keep it moist, thus preventing wrinkling. Just massage it in.

ALMOND OIL: This has also been used for thousands of years in the same way as olive oil.

WITCH HAZEL: Easily available from supermarkets and health shops, witch hazel is excellent for skin conditions in general and can be added to water to make a facial wash.

HORSE CHESTNUT: Research shows that horse chestnut is effective against wrinkles. Ask at your health shop for a cream containing it and apply as directed. (See Horse chestnut, page 187.)

ROSEMARY: Rosemary contains many anti-ageing properties generally, so it's a good one for your diet. Look for rosemary tea or make your own from the dried herb by adding a teaspoonful to water. (See Rosemary, page 226.)

COLD WATER: I always remember one woman who had lovely fresh skin, telling me that her secret was cold water, and having done a little research on it, as well as trying it myself, I would actually recommend it (if you live in an area with soft water, that is). Washing your face in it, twice a day, is a very good way of keeping the skin tight. Don't use soap. Just dip in and do it. Then towel dry.

A WORD OF CAUTION: Please refer to the individual instructions for each remedy. If you should experience any problem with using a particular cream, then stop.

INTERESTING FACT: The Victorian beauty suggestion for getting rid of wrinkles is to massage and pummel the skin in order to tone up the muscles underneath. I bet they had a few black eyes.

A-Z of Remedies and Therapies

Acupressure

WHAT IS IT? Acupressure is a therapy that has been around for rather a long time. In fact, it is the 'granddaddy' of them all in many ways, even outdoing acupuncture in the age game. In many cultures acupressure is used to relieve pain and stress. In China, from where it originates, it is used just as we use first aid. That is, for everything from colds to hangovers! And by this or that family member on others.

HOW DOES IT WORK? In traditional Chinese medicine, health is viewed as a constantly changing flow of energy. So if that flow is disturbed in any way, then sickness results. Typically the aim is to release blocked energy by pressing on certain acupoints, which sit on the energy channels. Once the energy is flowing the body should be in a better position to start healing itself.

WHAT DOES IT HELP IN PARTICULAR? Acupressure is especially good for relieving pain and muscle tension. Migraine and back pain sufferers in particular find it useful. So do people with chronic sinusitis. It is also commonly used for morning sickness and motion sickness.

HOW LONG SHOULD A COURSE OF TREATMENT LAST? Depending on the condition treatments can last anything from 15 minutes to an hour and afterwards you might feel a little achy rather than sore. The amount of actual sessions you need depends on the problem. It can be six, eight or more. Sometimes it happens that the problem you have isn't responding to treatment on a particular day, however, so in some ways that is a treatment 'wasted', so to speak.

HOW DO I GO ABOUT GETTING THIS TREATMENT? Ask first at your health centre or shop for a list of practitioners in the area. Often acupressure is linked with Shiatsu and massage. Other alternatives are to learn the technique yourself from books or videos. But if you do, please pay attention to the cautionary note.

A WORD OF CAUTION: Because acupressure involves massage, it is important that you are comfortable with your practitioner. If you have any doubts at all, then find someone else. Also, remember to tell your practitioner if you have a tumour, or are pregnant, as certain pressure points must be avoided. Open wounds, bruises, scars, broken bones or varicose veins should not be pressed and you should certainly avoid acupressure if you have a lung or kidney disorder, a contagious disease, infectious skin disease, or a serious heart condition.

INTERESTING FACT: Acupressure was first developed in China over 5,000 years ago, probably out of the natural human instinct to hold a part that is sore.

Acupuncture

WHAT IS IT? I think this is a therapy we all enjoy a bit of a giggle about – the idea of looking a bit like the man in the ad for the film *The Hellraiser* – a sort of human pincushion. The practice of inserting needles into certain points of the body to relieve various conditions, has been around for thousands of years and isn't at all as painful as you would think. Some people even fall asleep during a session, so it can't be that bad! Acupuncture is a big part of Chinese medicine, part of the philosophy that views health as a changing flow of energy. It works by regulating the imbalances in the flow that result in disease.

HOW DOES IT WORK? Well, now for the gory part! To strengthen the flow of energy and/or remove blockages, the acupuncturist inserts tiny, wafer-thin needles just under the skin at certain points along the energy channels. Anything from one to fifteen needles can be used and these are left in for 15 to 40 minutes. Some acupuncturists sometimes send a weak electrical current through the needles. Don't worry, it is very weak. You're not going to jolt from the chair or anything! Some people experience a tingling in their limbs, others say they feel a little uncomfortable, while some don't notice anything at all. While the needles are in, the nerves are being stimulated and, rather like a telegraph system, messages are being sent to a primitive part of the brain and the pituitary gland. These parts then 'telegraph' back, sending chemicals that block pain signals. Research has shown that acupuncture does alter the circulation, increasing blood flow to the area that relays pain.

WHAT DOES IT HELP IN PARTICULAR? Acupuncture is good for nausea caused by chemotherapy, post-operative pain and morning sickness. Because it can relieve pain, it can help headache, back pain and arthritis. While it cannot cure these conditions, it is also useful for asthma sufferers and for stroke rehabilitation.

HOW LONG SHOULD A COURSE OF TREATMENT LAST? A session generally lasts up to an hour and can take place once or twice a week. The amount of sessions needed depends very much on the condition and how it responds to therapy.

HOW DO I GO ABOUT GETTING THIS TREATMENT? Initially you should ask your doctor for a therapist.

A WORD OF CAUTION: If you have diabetes, then the practitioner should insert the needles with a great deal of care, as even a small cut can lead to a bad infection. People on anticoagulants should consult their doctor before taking this treatment, as should pregnant women. Although acupuncture can help morning sickness, stimulation of the points near the abdomen can cause premature labour and possibly miscarriage. So be sure to tell the acupuncturist if you think you may be pregnant. Also, tell them if you have a pacemaker fitted, as electrical stimulation of the needles could certainly cause problems, as could magnets. Lastly, certain contagious diseases and hepatitis B can be passed from infected needles, so please make sure that the therapist you choose uses disposable needles.

INTERESTING FACT: There are over 1,000 acupuncture points on the body.

Alexander Technique

WHAT IS IT? It may sound like some kind of strange sexual position but the Alexander Technique is a method of improving posture, letting go of tension and moving with better ease. It was 'discovered' by an Australian actor whose career was on a downward spiral because of persistent hoarseness. He looked in the mirror one day, saw that he tensed his neck when he spoke and realised that this was the cause. When he changed his posture, hey presto, the condition vanished. The rest, as they say, is history.

HOW DOES IT WORK? The Alexander Technique is based on the belief that if the relationship between a person's neck, head and spine is correct, then their health will be good. An incorrect position can cause tension and pain. At a session you will be encouraged to breathe freely, to relax your neck muscles. Through gentle touch and verbal instruction your limbs will be stretched out and repositioned. You might even find you're 'floating on air', to some extent. Things that were off balance will be pointed out to you, so that you see what you're doing wrong. Bad habits will be replaced by good habits, easing pressure on certain muscles.

WHAT DOES IT HELP IN PARTICULAR? Because it looks at posture, the Alexander Technique is very good if you are suffering chronic neck and back pain. It's also useful for arthritis, migraine and anxiety. Pregnant women, too, feel that it helps them to cope with the changes to their body, while athletes and dancers often find it can help them maintain their form as they play or dance and help them to prevent wear and tear on the body as well as injuries.

HOW LONG SHOULD A COURSE OF TREATMENT LAST? Most sessions last about 45 minutes and the number of sessions really depends on how well you do. In some instances, people can learn to use their bodies more effectively with as little as six sessions.

HOW DO I GO ABOUT GETTING THIS TREATMENT? You can learn this privately on a one-to-one basis or go as part of a group. Sessions don't always come cheaply, however, so it must be something you really feel will help. To find a practitioner, you can contact the Society of Teachers of the Alexander Technique (STAT), at www.stat.org.uk, who will put you in touch with a teacher in your area.

A WORD OF CAUTION: When taught by a proper practitioner, this technique is safe for everyone.

INTERESTING FACT: Needless to say, Mr Alexander was soon able to give up the day job and spend his time teaching his technique as well as writing books about it. Today the technique he founded way back in 1896 is taught all over the world and used in many stage schools.

Aloe Vera

The Africans take the credit for finding this wonderfully versatile product. A fairly sinister looking plant in its spiky form, most of the goodness comes from the individual leaves where we obtain liquid, gel and latex (left over as a sticky substance once the liquid has been evaporated).

DETOXING: This is the main use I've had personally and have advised dozens of times to my clients. Aloe Vera juice is not only easily obtained but is a pleasant and hugely effective drink. By way of some examples, I have recommended Aloe Vera juice to clients suffering from Irritable Bowel Syndrome and a few other bowel disorders, such as constipation.

CONSTIPATION: Aloe Vera capsules are easily obtained from good health stores and, following manufacturers' instructions, constipation can be cured within 48 hours. This remedy should be discontinued after ten days maximum.

MINOR CUTS AND BURNS: Aloe Vera gel – something my medicine cabinet is never without – is a great pain reliever when applied to the skin three times a day.

MOUTH ULCERS: When applied to the affected area, Aloe Vera gel can be effective in reducing swelling and pain.

PSORIASIS: Aloe Vera creams can be rubbed on the affected patch (or patches) of skin for what I've found to be a successful outcome.

COLIC: The root of the Aloe Vera plant has been found to be successful in reducing colic and other stomach-related problems.

A WORD OF CAUTION: As with all burns and wounds, if severe, aloe gel, like any other substance applied, may in fact result in blistering and can therefore slow down the healing process. Laxative use can worsen constipation and can result in dependency. The latex form of Aloe Vera should not be used by children or by pregnant women. Long-term use of latex aloe may result in potassium deficiency.

INTERESTING FACTS: One of my clients used Aloe Vera juice to detox her somewhat alcohol-abused body and subsequently drinks nothing but Aloe Vera juice along with other fruit juices.

Amino acids

The amino acids might sound like something you'd find in a teenager's CD rack. They're actually where the body gets its protein from. Very necessary for human growth and all that. And they come in two types: essential and non-essential. The non-essential amino acids can always be manufactured by the body if it's not getting them. But the essential can't. These have to come from foods. So it's important that you're eating properly and in particular that you have these acids in your diet. Just because you're all grown up now, don't think you don't need them. It doesn't stop there. Amino acids are vital for repair and maintenance of all organs, glands and muscles, certain bodily fluids – just all kinds of things. Fruit – in particular, apples, pears and apricots – is a good source. So are vegetables, watercress, lentils and soy beans. In addition to this, however, actual supplements can help with certain diseases. Here are a few examples.

HEART DISEASE: Amino acids may help fight heart disease and alleviate associated pains in the legs.

STROKE: Certain amino acids, taken in supplement form, may help to fight stroke by lowering blood pressure.

BOOSTING THE IMMUNE SYSTEM: Because they give the body protein, amino acid supplements can help boost the immune system, helping to prevent you from getting diseases.

HERPES: Lysine – one of the acids – is very good for treating cold sores. Either start eating plenty of the foodstuffs mentioned above, or take a supplement. Lysine supplements should be taken with water, not milk.

A WORD OF CAUTION: Well, there are one or two! Firstly, you have to know what you're doing if you take supplements. That's because there are all kinds of amino acids and they're used for different things. You have to be sure you're using the appropriate one, so this might be something to discuss with your doctor. If you are pregnant or have a serious illness, don't take supplements without consulting them anyway, although of course it is safe to up your intake of the foodstuffs mentioned. Lysine should not be taken with milk. If you take supplements, don't overdose on them, thinking 'the more the merrier'. Excessive amounts can lead to vomiting. Just follow the instructions and never take them for months on end. They're really intended for short-term use.

INTERESTING FACT: Supplements are thought to reduce sugar cravings!

Ancient Chinese medicine

WHAT IS IT? Although it's very much in vogue right now, Chinese medicine has in fact been around for hundreds of years – 2,500 to be precise, which is rather a lot, I would say, wouldn't you? As to what it involves, well that's rather a great deal too! Down the years it has evolved to cover many things – acupuncture and massage to name but two. Then there are herbal remedies, dietary principles, Tai Chi and Qigong.

HOW DOES IT WORK? Although we might joke about the yin and the yang, practitioners of Chinese medicine take it very seriously. Yin and yang are not two strange-sounding Scottish gentlemen, second cousins twice removed, but opposing qualities which must be properly balanced for good health to result. Then there's the five Chinese elements: wood, fire, earth, metal and water, which practitioners believe our internal organs are related to. Lastly there's the thorough evaluation of the body to determine what part needs the most support and what this support will be. And while all this sounds very airy-fairy and as if we're flying in the wind with our water, earth and fire, it's actually much more sophisticated than that. In many instances, certain conditions can be improved by changing a person's diet, while more physical problems can benefit from treatments such as massage. Any medical mixture that is prescribed is sure to be carefully formulated from many sources with your condition in mind.

WHAT DOES IT HELP IN PARTICULAR? Because Chinese medicine is such a 'wide umbrella', and includes a number of therapies, it can help many things. Some of the therapies are already mentioned elsewhere. Actual herbal remedies can treat flu, cold, migraine, dermatitis and irritable bowel syndrome.

HOW LONG SHOULD A COURSE OF TREATMENT LAST? Where herbal medicine is involved, this will depend very much on the ailment. Colds and flu, for example, can be treated quickly. If it's something that's more of a problem, then you might have to take a remedy for a few weeks before seeing an improvement.

HOW DO I GO ABOUT GETTING THIS TREATMENT? Since many health shops carry lists of therapists, ask there first. In some of the larger cities, practitioners can be found nestling between the high street shops. Just remember to check out their background first. It takes years to study Chinese medicine. So look for one who knows all the processes.

A WORD OF CAUTION: Remember not to take anything that you may have an allergy to. So if the remedy you have been given disagrees with you, then try something else instead. Don't expect miracles right away. Herbal tonics can take time. But if your condition shows absolutely no sign of improvement after weeks of trying, and you haven't seen a doctor, then you should do so.

INTERESTING FACT: Although Chinese medicine has been around for hundreds of years, and indeed was brought to the rest of the world by traders and missionaries, it declined in China, until the government realised it was a good way to improve the population's healthcare.

Antiseptic

Unless you're someone who's been living on another planet all their days, then you're bound to know what antiseptic is and that it's ideal for killing germs, cleansing wounds and cuts, and reducing inflammation where the wound has become septic and has started to give trouble. Obviously, all kinds of creams are readily available that can soon go to work, but there are also many herbal alternatives which you might like to try, too. The ones I recommend are:

CALENDULA: You can either steep the flowers in hot water to make a rinse for cuts, or look for a calendula cream at your health shop. Calendula contains many antiseptic compounds. (See Calendula, page 144.)

COMFREY: Again, very useful as an antiseptic. You can find skin creams containing it at your health shop. (See Comfrey, page 154.)

TEA TREE OIL: This oil has been used for hundreds of years as an antiseptic. You can buy a bottle of oil from your health shop. It's a good one to keep handy in case you ever need it. Then you can dab it on the affected area. (See Tea tree oil, page 233.)

MARSH MALLOW: Poultices of marsh mallow have been used for hundreds of years to treat wounds. It contains many antiseptic qualities. Ask at your health shop for preparations containing it. (See Marsh mallow, page 200.)

GOLDENSEAL: This is very good for reducing inflammation and treating cuts. Ask at your health shop for products containing it.

CLOVE: I'm sure this is one you'll know well from your childhood and also from visits to the dentist. Oil of clove is also a painkiller. It's very good for cuts and inflammations.

GARLIC: Yes, garlic is one I don't hesitate to recommend. Moreover, it's one we all tend to have in the kitchen. If you have the powdered kind, or can cut up a clove, then you can make an antiseptic paste with a little water and spread it on the affected area. (See Garlic, page 174.)

EUCALYPTUS: Traditionally used as an antiseptic and disinfectant, this is one of my favourites. One I also keep handy just in case. (See Eucalyptus, page 164.)

WITCH HAZEL: This is excellent for many skin conditions and very easily obtainable from supermarkets. (See Witch hazel, page 252.)

A WORD OF CAUTION: Please refer to theindividual remedy to see what is best for you. Calendula, for example, won't suit you if you suffer from hayfever, and garlic can sometimes cause irritation. Also, never take any oils. They are intended for external use only and can be highly poisonous if swallowed.

INTERESTING FACT: The Greeks and Romans burned their antiseptic herbs in censers and carried them into the streets to ward off infection. I bet their streets smelled better than ours at that time!

Aromatherapy

WHAT IS IT? Rather as the name suggests, this is something of a 'smell therapy'. If you ever had a cold as a child and were made to inhale a steaming basin of something or other to help clear it, then you'll have a rough idea of what it is. Smell is perhaps the most acute of our senses, often triggering memories and responses from other parts of our systems. Aromatherapy takes this one stage further by matching essential oils from plants to certain conditions.

HOW DOES IT WORK? Aromatherapy can be used in a number of ways, by adding the oils to a bath, inhaling the scents, and by massaging the oils into the skin. Therapists believe that the oils then work either emotionally, reminding you of happy times, or physically by stimulating the immune or nervous system. The oils that are used are essential ones, rather than just ones scented with herbs, as many bath and beauty products are.

WHAT DOES IT HELP IN PARTICULAR? Aromatherapy is not a cure in itself, obviously, or we'd all have our noses stuck in a burner all day long, inhaling all these wonderful oils! It can, however, benefit existing conditions such as colds, flu, insomnia, tension, anxiety, muscle pains, depression and migraine. And, basically, it's horses for courses. Certain oils for certain conditions.

HOW LONG SHOULD A COURSE OF TREATMENT LAST? This depends on whether you are simply buying oil to inhale either from a burner, or on a hanky, by sniffing the scent, or by placing them in a basin of steaming water. Some people place the oils in a bath, others go to a trained aromatherapist who massages the oils into the skin. So the length of time it takes for this treatment is very variable and depends on how often you use it.

HOW DO I GO ABOUT GETTING THIS TREATMENT? There has never been an easier time for 'getting' aromatherapy. So many shops and chemists are bursting at the seams with essential oils, all you have to do is buy a burner, some oil, a night light and hey presto! You must make sure, however, that the oil you burn is the one for your condition. Lavender oil, for example, won't relieve your cold but it could help you relax. So ask when you buy, or read up on it first. Trained aromatherapists do exist if you want to see one. Generally, they are also trained in massage. Ask at your health shop for a list of them.

A WORD OF CAUTION: Well, there are quite a few actually. People assume, 'Oh this is just from some herb, it's okay to burn or chuck in the bath, or whatever.' Well let me tell you, it's not. When I was new to this I was lucky to step out of the bath alive, after misreading the instructions on one herbal oil! Not exactly, I am joking of course, but I did come out clutching the sides. I had fever, palpitations and then lay in a cold sweat for the next six hours. So you must be careful, be very careful – to paraphrase a well-known movie moment. Read everything properly and obey all instructions to the letter. Never take any oil, and if you're using it on the skin, dilute it with olive oil and put a little on the skin first and wait 24 hours to check you're not allergic. If you have asthma, consult your doctor first, as certain oils can trigger bronchial spasms. Also, unless you really know what you're doing, it's best to avoid using aromatherapy if you're pregnant and to my knowledge it tells you this on the instructions for particular bath products. Certain oils can trigger miscarriage or hurt the baby. It's also important not to persist in smelling oils that bring back bad memories.

INTERESTING FACT: Plant oils have been used for thousands of years for therapeutic purposes. The actual term Aromatherapy was coined in the 1920s and the therapy fully developed in the 1950s.

Aspirin

Even before the aspirin, as we all know it and love it, was developed, the compounds that it contains could be found in certain herbs. Meadowsweet and willow bark in particular, were used both for colds and cooling the fevered brow, and if you want to be very strict about this and try a herbal aspirin, then you will certainly find one. What I would like to talk about here, however, is just good old plain aspirin – great for so many things and very easily available. Often, with so many other remedies on the market, it's easy to forget its pain-relieving qualities.

FEVER: Aspirin is very good for reducing the kind of mild fever associated with colds or flu. By mild I am meaning a temperature between 99 °F and 101 °F. Obviously if it is higher than that you must consult a doctor. Remember that, up to a point, a fever is the body's way of getting rid of poisons. If you have the cold and it has led to a higher than usual temperature then you would certainly find aspirin helpful.

HEADACHES: Again, a couple of aspirins help soothe a sore head, provided it's not of the splitting migraine variety. Since cold and flu sufferers tend to get a headache, often because of blocked sinuses, it can be doing several jobs at the same time so to speak. Aspirin contains compounds that help clear catarrh, thus getting rid of blocked noses and clearing sore heads.

MINOR ACHES: I take aspirin myself if I've got a sore anything! I don't see the point of going about with something that's sore and making matters worse by tensing the muscles round about the ache. If you have a minor ache, pain or strain, then an aspirin can help. Again, cold and flu sufferers can find relief from aching bones.

RHEUMATISM: Aspirin is still reckoned to be one of the best helps for rheumatics. Many sufferers swear that taking one every morning not only helps with the aches and pains but also seems to stop the condition getting worse.

THINNING BLOOD: As with rheumatic sufferers, there are a number of elderly people who put their longevity down to taking an aspirin each day. Too many to ignore, I would say! Trials have shown that aspirin does actually thin the blood, thus cutting down the risk of strokes. If you consider yourself at risk, then this is one remedy that is definitely worth pursuing.

A WORD OF CAUTION: While aspirin is on the whole safe, doing much more good than harm, some people can be allergic to the substances that are in it and cases of gastrorintestinal bleeding caused by asprin have been recorded. If you are one of these people, then I'm afraid this isn't for you. Nor is a herbal alternative, because these contain the same compounds that aspirin is made from. Also, remember that you should not give aspirin to children with colds, flu or chickenpox because there is a chance that they might develop a condition that can damage the liver and brain. This is a small chance only but worth considering all the same.

INTERESTING FACT: Aspirin was 'discovered' in the eighteenth century when a British minister tried to find a cheap substitute for cinchona bark, which was used to treat malaria and other fevers. He used willow bark instead. The rest, as they say, is history!

Bach Flower Remedies

WHAT IS IT? The Bach Flower Remedies were developed in the 1920s and 1930s by Dr Edward Bach. He believed that illness was a symptom of emotional imbalance and, rather tired of conventional medicine, he set out to find plants that could relieve certain conditions. Negative emotions reduce the body's natural resistance to disease, said Dr Bach, predisposing certain people to particular illnesses – something that has since been determined by scientific studies. By testing his remedies on himself, Dr Bach discovered, for example, that mustard could get rid of gloom.

HOW DOES IT WORK? Bach Flower Remedies won't treat a condition, but they aim to try to get rid of the emotional stress that is stopping the body from healing itself. They also work to counteract your fears about an illness. Before he died, Dr Bach had worked his way through 38 remedies in all. So that accounts for quite a lot of illnesses! With Bach Flowers the appropriate remedy is generally administered as a tincture, one or two drops being placed under the tongue, or put in water and sipped. In some instances the tincture can be put in a bath. As your state of mind improves the remedy can be adjusted.

WHAT DOES IT HELP IN PARTICULAR? In addition to generally helping the body react more positively, Bach Flower Remedies are very good for all stress-related conditions, depression, headache, insomnia and anxiety. They can also help with chronic pain and PMT. Bach's Rescue Remedy, which can be bought from health shops, is one of the best things for treating shock.

HOW LONG SHOULD A COURSE OF TREATMENT LAST? Generally if you are choosing Bach Flower Remedies then the treatment will last till the emotional state is relieved. This can be after one session or 60! It just depends on your state of mind and how deeply rooted the problem is.

HOW DO I GO ABOUT GETTING THIS TREATMENT? If you want you can go to a health shop where they are widely available and ask for a pamphlet to help you decide what one you need, though you might find there's a bit of trial and error in doing this. Or you can consult a herbalist, homeopath, aromatherapist or other practitioner trained in selecting the essence. Someone who really knows what they're doing can make the remedy up as prescribed by Dr Bach himself.

A WORD OF CAUTION: Because the Remedies are alcohol based, they should be avoided by pregnant women and alcoholics. Also, please remember that, although they are safe on the whole, they are not a substitute for medical care if that's what your condition requires. If you've been prescribed other drugs, you must keep taking them.

INTERESTING FACT: Dr Bach's name was actually pronounced 'Botch'. I'm not going to comment on that one!

Basil

I'm rather fond of this herb. It's a wonderful culinary flavouring, especially on pizzas and pastas, as well as smelling not too unpleasant. Basil does have other uses too, however. Other cultures have used it traditionally and extensively as a medical herb, one that is useful for curing certain ailments. You might like to try doing the same by adding basil to your diet. I can't think of a nicer way.

Basil is easily obtainable in dried form from your supermarket. Even better, you can always grow your own.

HALITOSIS: Basil is good for curing bad breath. If it's in your food generally, it's improving the digestion. You can also try putting a spoonful in a cup of boiling water, letting it sit for ten minutes, straining, then using the cooled basil as a mouthwash to rinse your mouth. It should certainly help. Just make sure the liquid is properly cooled before you do this. I don't think it would help matters if you burnt your mouth!

HEADACHE: You can try adding a spoonful of basil to your tea if you have a headache, letting it sit and straining before drinking. Traditionally, basil was used for this purpose.

WARTS: Basil was also traditionally used to cure warts. If you have one, you can try rubbing the fresh leaves on, every day. (See Warts, page 112.)

EMPHYSEMA: Basil contains compounds that make it useful as an expectorant. If you suffer from this condition, then adding it regularly to your food can't do any harm. It's delicious when sprinkled on onions with a sprinkling of garlic powder and chilli, then fried in olive oil, for pizza toppings. If you add a little bacon, even better.

A WORD OF CAUTION: None that I can think of.

INTERESTING FACT: In India and Africa, basil is used as an insect repellent. All you have to do is rub on the leaves!

Beta-carotene

Trying to ensure that your diet is healthy, is one of the best preventative measures against disease and a healthy diet should have a reasonable amount of fruit and vegetables in it – something that, let's be honest, is sometimes easier said than done. This strange-sounding antioxidant is a pigment that gives certain fruits and vegetables their red, orange and yellow colour. Once eaten, the body converts it to vitamin A. But beta-carotene has other uses too.

Presently scientists are exploring its potential for treating male infertility and psoriasis. It is also thought that some of the properties in beta-carotene can slow the progress of Alzheimer's disease, as well as preventing heart disease, certain cancers, and boosting the immune system generally – something that makes for better health all round – so it's well worth getting better acquainted with its properties.

Beta-carotene is at its most effective when taken as a supplement, particularly when combined with other antioxidants such as alpha-carotene. You should avoid taking supplements if you smoke or suffer from liver or kidney disease, a sluggish thyroid or an eating disorder. If this is the case then try to make a conscious effort to eat more carrots – a good source – or try a glass of carrot juice instead!

A WORD OF CAUTION: Smokers should avoid beta-carotene as some studies have shown a likely increase in the risk of lung cancer unless you take both beta-carotene and vitamin E. Apart from that, it would appear that there are no proven side effects to beta-carotene. However, overdoing it (usually exceeding 60 mg per day) can cause a discoloration on the skin.

INTERESTING FACTS: I think we all tend to think beta-carotene is found only in carrots or other orange vegetables. However, some of our greens contain beta-carotene too. A client of mine found using beta-carotene helped wean her off alcohol. Tests underway right now are hoping to find evidence that beta-carotene may prevent heart illness, slow down Alzheimer's disease and help with male infertility. Watch this space!

Bilberry

These dark blue berries are sometimes overlooked in the health stakes, although I'm sure we've all heard of bilberry pies, jam and muffins, which I confess I go weak kneed about! They are, however, beneficial for treating certain conditions. If you're a sufferer of any of these then think about adding bilberries to your diet. You can't go wrong. Even if you're not, bilberries generally do our insides good, so get eating. What a pleasant way to keep healthy!

ANGINA: Bilberry is good for lowering the cholesterol, so eating them can do no harm if you suffer from this condition. In addition to this they open the blood vessels and lower blood pressure.

MENSTRUAL CRAMPS: Many herbalists suggest taking bilberry extract for this condition. The compounds in bilberry have muscle relaxant properties that can help ease away painful cramps. The recommended dose is 20–40 mg, three times a day. Ask at your health food shop. If they can't help, try eating a bowl of fresh bilberries.

ULCERS: Bilberry contains a compound called anthocyanoside – rather a mouthful to pronounce. Far simpler to know that this compound offers protection against ulcers, by stimulating the mucus that protects the stomach wall. If you're a sufferer at all, then make a conscious effort to add bilberries to your diet and let them do their work.

DIARRHOEA: Dried bilberry helps relieve diarrhoea because it contains pectin.

AVAILABILITY: Bilberries can be purchased at the fruit counter of many supermarkets, or ask at your health store for bilberry extract. Fresh bilberries are delicious and personally I can't think of a better way of keeping fit!

A WORD OF CAUTION: So long as you stick to jams, extracts, capsules, etc., you should find no side effects. Not that you are every likely to, but I'd avoid eating the leaves of bilberry as they can be poisonous. As with any herb or supplement in my book, always consult the manufacturer's guidelines just to be on the safe side.

INTERESTING FACT: Eighteenth-century herbalists used the antioxidant properties in bilberry as a mouthwash. Pilots flying at night say their vision is vastly improved after using bilberry extracts. This was discovered initially after they ate toast with bilberry jam! Opticians may find themselves becoming extinct if there is enough proof in the fact that bilberry, when taken wisely, can improve eyesight – especially at night. In olden times, bilberry was used long before insulin was discovered.

Black cohosh

This amazing and therapeutic supplement is best known for its abilities to help the female gender. It has other abilities too but primarily it is good for ailments ranging from menstrual cramps to the symptoms of the menopause, for which it can be used as a substitute HRT.

Black cohosh is a flower first discovered and used by women at the beginning of the twentieth century. It became more and more popular when it began to help women with a whole range of 'women's problems', such as, as I've said, cramps, heavy bleeding, hot flushes. For some reason there was some controversy over black cohosh but it has come back with a vengeance, helping with not only women's problems but also pain relief and as an anti-inflammatory.

MENSTRUAL CRAMPS: Unless you're a woman, you can't fully understand the extent of this ghastly pain. I've heard many women complain that they are not taken seriously because this is, and I quote, 'only a woman's problem', with the undertone that it isn't serious. Anyone suffering from menstrual cramps will know just how serious they can be. Black cohosh is not only used for pain relief but is also renowned for it's anti-inflammatory abilities. Therefore, this wonder herbal drug is perfect for many women's problems.

NEURALGIA: Black cohosh can ease the pain of this dreadful illness, not only because of its pain-killing ability but also as it contains a mild sedative. Any kind of tooth or gum problem is awful, so if you are unable to sleep due to the pain, black cohosh is, once again, a great supplement.

BONES: Any ailment involving the joints, such as arthritis, rheumatism and osteoporosis can be eased by using black cohosh.

TEA INFUSION: Ask at your local health store for dried root of black cohosh. Pour a cup of water over a teaspoonful of the dried root and bring to the boil. Allow this to simmer for ten minutes, cool and drink, up to three times a day. It is advisable to add a teaspoonful of honey as it has a fairly bitter taste. It can also be bought in capsule and tincture form.

WHOOPING COUGH: Due to black cohosh's ability to reduce spasms, some reports suggest it is beneficial for this complaint.

A WORD OF CAUTION: Black cohosh is thought to be largely safe even for children but it should be avoided by pregnant or lactating women. Some studies have also shown it can interfere with the Pill and so you should establish whether or not you are able to combine the two. To avoid stomach upset, you should take black cohosh with meals. Use with caution and stick to the manufacturer's advised dosage.

INTERESTING FACTS: Although thought to be unsafe for pregnant women, black cohosh has been found to be of great benefit during childbirth itself. During the 1800s, American doctors used black cohosh to reduce fever.

Blackberry

Blackberry or bramble is common throughout Europe and America and is characterised by its prickly, long trailing stem, which is absolutely no fun to get close to! So, unless you want to be looking up the cure for nasty scratches, do be careful if you go picking your own.

Blackberries very often grow wild, so it's great to go brambling in autumn and pick the fruit for jam, if you live in a country area. The distinct, raspberry-like berries are good for other things besides, as are the leaves, especially when mixed with the aforementioned raspberry

DIARRHOEA: Blackberry leaves mixed with those of the raspberry are good for easing this condition. You can try making a tea by pouring hot water on two teaspoons of blackberry and two of raspberry leaf. Or you can keep some blackberry tea bags handy in your cupboard for when the need arises. It's always a good idea to have a stock of things in your home, so that you can treat conditions as they arise, instead of having to rush out to the chemists every time. Most supermarkets that have a herbal tea bar include blackberry, as do local health stores. If raspberry is included, so much the better. Three cups a day should ease things considerably.

TONSILLITIS: A painful condition, tonsillitis can be eased by taking blackberry root and persimmon. Ask at your local health store for a combination extract.

A WORD OF CAUTION: I can think of none, so again, read the label before using blackberry.

INTERESTING FACT: Early American settlers used blackberry root for tonsillitis. The tannin apparently worked wonders.

Bran

Bran is one of those foods that is easy to take for granted, because it's readily available, cheap and something our mothers probably swore by. You know, I've even heard it said that cakes made with bran can help you diet. Supposedly it's because they're very filling. I've never tried it myself. So who am I to scoff! Here are some of the things it *is* good for, however.

CONSTIPATION: This is probably one of the best-known uses of bran. Two tablespoonfuls every morning were recommended to deal with this problem. And sprinkling it on a cereal was suggested for generally keeping things regular. Nowadays of course, many cereals are bran-based, so to speak, and people find taking them is an easy way to keep healthy. Then there is bran bread, which, for a number of reasons, including providing fibre, is better than white. Regular sufferers might find that the swap would be very beneficial. Should your constipation continue, however, or should you suddenly find yourself suffering from it for no good reason, having previously had no trouble, please consult your doctor.

PLEURISY: Bran tea is an old folk remedy for this condition and one you can make yourself, if you have bran to hand. Just boil one tablespoonful of bran in a litre of water. Skim, strain and add a tablespoonful of honey. Obviously bran has other effects so you might not want to drink too much of it! But you could certainly try a cup each day to help give your body the strength and energy to fight off this infection.

ACHING JOINTS: Traditionally, bran poultices were all the rage when it came to dealing with certain rheumatic conditions. Sciatica and gout too – although I'm not certain that I would want to sit with a vinegar, bran and garlic soaked cloth on my foot if I had gout. Still, who knows, if I was desperate I might change my mind!

INFLAMED SKIN: If you have patches of inflamed skin, then bran and ivy can help. Just chop up a handful of ordinary ivy leaves and mix them with six tablespoons of bran and a little warm water to make a paste. Then apply to the affected area.

A WORD OF CAUTION: Unless you have some kind of food allergy that means you can't eat it, bran is very good for you and there are very definite benefits to the digestive health of those who do take it.

INTERESTING FACT: Bran was traditionally used for feeding animals until its benefits to humans became clear.

Brazil nuts

Not only is there a lot of coffee in Brazil but a lot of nuts too. The Brazil nut, however, is the very edible seed of a South American tree, harvested from January to June and very useful for a variety of ailments, because of its antioxidant properties. Even just munching one or two a day can help in a variety of ways. For example, their essential trace oils, might help slow cataracts. Just don't go eating too many more than that. Nuts in general are terrible for piling on the pounds. It's not a diet book I want to be writing next!

ALZHEIMER'S DISEASE: Because Brazil nuts contain high quantities of lecithin, a substance that's good for the brain, taking them on a regular basis could help sharpen the memory, thus lessening the chances of developing this condition. (See Alzheimer's disease, page 14.)

ARTHRITIS: While it would simply not be feasible to eat the amount of Brazil nuts that would be as effective as a standard dose of some arthritic medicines – we would get very fat indeed – Brazil nuts do contain pain-relieving and anti-inflammatory properties. Including them in your diet therefore, on a regular or daily basis, over a period of time, could help act preventatively, with regard to this condition.

PSORIASIS: As well as lecithin, Brazil nuts contain vitamin E and selenium. In the Amazon, people use this oil to treat skin conditions. Eating Brazil nuts regularly may help people with psoriasis. It's well worth a try. However, it is also possible to buy Brazil nut oil at health food stores and rub it on the affected skin in order to relieve the itching associated with this condition.

A WORD OF CAUTION: Obviously, those with any kind of allergy to nuts should steer well clear of the advice offered on this page.

INTERESTING FACT: The playwright Brandon Thomas must have liked Brazil nuts. In his play *Charlie's Aunt*, his favourite punch line was, 'She's from Brazil, where the nuts come from.'

Burdock

This is one ancient remedy I'm sure most of you have heard of. In olden times (not that long ago) a common remedy was burdock and dandelion in the form of a juice drink. Now we see it available in a few forms from tincture to capsules. It's known in the trade as 'the purifier of blood', which means it is good for a vast range of ailments. Burdock roots can be found quite easily in fruit markets etc., but many people are put off because, in root form, it looks dirty. This should not put you off, as you can easily wash the root. In looks it resembles a carrot, except that it is darker, and brown in colour rather than orange. Burdock is also a great way of boosting our magnesium and potassium intake. Identifying the plant in the wild is fairly easy as it's one of the 'sticky plants' – meaning that if you brush past it, it will stick to your clothes.

Burdock can be successfully used in a whole array of ailments, ranging from facial spots to tonsillitis, from arthritis to measles.

SKIN DISORDERS: Due to its purifying qualities, burdock is brilliant for the skin, eczema, boils, or just for overall good skin texture.

PSORIASIS: Again, due to its purifying qualities, burdock also works as an anti-inflammatory. It is therefore also good for gout, arthritis and any kind of swelling, even water retention, as it's a known diuretic.

BOWEL PROBLEMS: Not only recommended as a diuretic, burdock has also been known to act as a laxative.

COUGHS: Burdock tea is beneficial for most types of coughs. To use as a tea, place one piece of dried root into hot water, leave for 30 minutes.

INFECTION: The purifying qualities once again act wherever infection is lingering. Again, you can use burdock in tablet form, tincture form or as a tea.

A WORD OF CAUTION: As far as I have seen during my research on this book, no side effects have been documented. However, as always, follow the manufacturer's guidelines.

INTERESTING FACTS: Tests are currently being carried out into burdock tea as a prevention for cancer. There is as yet no known evidence of this. Using burdock root in broth allows an added flavour, one that is pleasant and fairly sweet. I received a letter from a reader saying she used burdock root on her seven-year-old son after he had been stung by a wasp.

Cabbage

Easily obtainable – you can grow your own – cabbage helps with many ailments. Indeed our mothers weren't too far wrong when they told us, 'Eat your greens,' although we probably didn't pay too much attention at the time, being far too busy wanting to eat lots of other things that were probably very bad for us! Cabbage contains several compounds that are good. If you don't care for the taste of it, you can always try putting it in soup or making a soup around it, with potatoes and celery. And there's always coleslaw of course, which is my favourite way of eating this vegetable.

ASTHMA: Cabbage contains some anti-asthmatic compounds. As a sufferer myself I am always on the lookout for ways to help keep things under control. That's why coleslaw is such a part of my diet. I'm not saying it works, and stops me having attacks altogether, just that it's one way of improving things for me. If you are a sufferer then you should look at your diet as a whole and try to include in it things that have these compounds.

MORNING SICKNESS: Cooked cabbage is an old time remedy for nausea and upset stomach, therefore it might help if you are pregnant and suffering from this quite horrible condition – the morning sickness that is, not the pregnancy! Certainly, it won't do any harm to you or the baby to increase your intake, and if it eases things, then so much the better.

ULCERS: Raw cabbage juice contains glutamine, which is very good for fighting ulcers. Unfortunately, it is rather disgusting to take.

Let's be honest, I wouldn't, unless you were going to twist my arm a bit or offer me a financial inducement! If you are a sufferer, however, it would be a good idea to make cabbage soup a regular part of your diet. As I've said before, every little helps. Eat healthy, stay healthy. Know your body and plan your diet accordingly.

OSTEOPOROSIS: Bones can be strengthened by eating cabbage. Many women over 50 suffer from this painful disease. So a daily helping of cabbage or coleslaw helps keep bones healthy. Cabbage contains boron, which raises oestrogen levels in the blood, levels that drop in older women.

INTERESTING FACTS: Lewis Carroll obviously did what his mother told him, or he wouldn't have written the line about 'cabbages and kings'.

Calcium

So here we are on the strong bones and teeth bit. The most abundant mineral in the human body. The one that is mainly found in bones and teeth. Some research shows that calcium may also be effective against heart attack, high blood pressure and PMS (pre-menstrual syndrome). We need to be sure we get enough. This of course starts with our diets. Good sources are green leafy vegetables, tinned salmon, sardines, and, of course, all dairy products – milk in particular. Of course, some people find it hard to incorporate these foodstuffs into their diets. Vegans in particular. But good calcium intake has so many benefits that if you can't you should perhaps consider taking supplements. Generally, calcium can help the following ailments.

OSTEOPOROSIS: This bone thinning disease, a dread of many women over a certain age, can be slowed, if not prevented, by making sure you have a good calcium intake. Studies of people over the age of 65 show that adding calcium-rich foods and supplements to their diets reduces the risk of bone loss. But don't wait till you're that age to think about this. Do it now and save yourself from 'shrinking' and developing a stooped posture.

BACK PAIN: Taking supplements or increasing your dietary intake can help strengthen your spine.

MIGRAINES: Calcium keeps the blood flowing throughout the body and may help stop these painful headaches.

HEARTBURN: Antacid tables containing calcium carbonate help relieve heartburn as well as neutralising gastric acid. Look for the ones with the carbonate, though – that's what does the trick.

PMS (PRE-MENSTRUAL SYNDROME): Some research indicates that low levels of calcium contribute to PMS. This isn't in all instances, but if you're a sufferer then it does no harm to rule this out. And if, in the process, you find the problem eases, then so much the better.

CRAMP: Too little calcium can also trigger muscle spasms. It's your body's way of telling you it wants more. If you suffer regularly it might be you're not getting enough calcium and should consider a supplement.

A WORD OF CAUTION: As a supplement, calcium is very easy to find and you should follow the dosage instructions. A recommended guide is about 1,000 mg a day for men and women between 19 and 50, and 1,200 mg a day for those between 50 and 70. Even if you go above that you still have to go very high for complications to set in, such as kidney stones. The body can't absorb any more than 500 mg of calcium at a time, so taking lots and lots isn't going to do you any good. It's also best to divide the daily dose, taking 500 mg in the morning, the rest at night. Supplements can, however, cause dehydration and sometimes constipation is the result. So drink lots of water. If you have kidney problems, or use thiazide diuretics, you must consult your doctor before taking supplements. Coupled with the diuretics they can cause high calcium levels, resulting in kidney failure. Something we don't want now do we? The same goes for thyroid disorders. Also, don't take calcium supplements within an hour of taking antibiotics. It lessens the efficiency of the drug.

INTERESTING FACT: Recent studies show that calcium might help prevent colon cancer. Certainly those with calcium-rich diets are less susceptible to it.

Calendula

You may be familiar with calendula. It's that big orange garden plant with all the petals that look not unlike those of a marigold. It's colour alone tells you it's full of carotenoids (see Beta-carotene, page 133). But it has other qualities too, as well as looking pretty in your garden!

BUNIONS: Some herbalists recommend calendula for this condition. (See Bunions, page 30.) While it won't reduce it, it can ease the pain. You can buy a salve or tincture from your health store and apply it, according to the instructions, when the bunion is sore or red. If it causes itching, as it can in some cases, discontinue use.

GINGIVITIS: Calendula has antibacterial properties, meaning it can kill germs, so you might just find it can help kill the germs that cause this condition and that you might be able to make up a mouthwash using the tincture. Or make a tea (See page 145), dip a cloth into it and apply it to the gums

SUNBURN: Calendula's many healing properties make it useful for healing burns. Look for a skin cream containing it in your health food shop and keep it handy just in case.

ULCERS: Clinical trials in Europe suggest that calendula may help reduce stomach inflammation, thus preventing ulcers from developing. It would also be good for treating gastritis and general stomach upset. Always remember, though, that if symptoms persist or take a turn for the worse and you are not happy, consult your doctor.

WOUNDS: Again, applying a cream with calendula in it can help heal sores.

SKIN TROUBLES: Problems such as eczema can respond to treatment with calendula, either as a cream, or when applied as a tincture.

AVAILABILITY: Ask at your health store for products containing calendula, such as tinctures or creams and use according to the instructions. You can place some drops of a tincture on a cloth to apply to certain skin conditions. Also, it is possible to make a tea by pouring a cup of boiling water over a flower. Allow it to steep for ten minutes, strain then drink.

A WORD OF CAUTION: While I personally have never experienced any problems in using or recommending calendula, I understand it can cause itching. If this happens, discontinue use. Calendula is a member of the ragwort family, so if you suffer from hayfever, it might be an idea to find something else.

INTERESTING FACT: Historically, calendula flowers were considered beneficial for the treatment of wounds.

Camomile

I'm very fond of camomile. I find it useful for lots of things and don't hesitate to recommend it to clients when I think it will do some good. As you can see, the list of ailments it can be used to help is long, so I won't hang about! Like many other herbal remedies, it has been used for centuries, although it's only in the last decade or so that its effects have been proven. These are the things I find it helps.

INSOMNIA: A cup of soothing camomile tea at bedtime can help you get to sleep and doesn't become addictive, so you've no worries there! (See Insomnia, page 73.)

HEARTBURN AND INDIGESTION: Camomile is effective for relieving both these conditions. Ask at your health shop for a tincture, which should have you right in no time.

PSORIASIS AND SKIN INFECTIONS: Camomile has a long history of being used to treat skin conditions. Psoriasis sufferers in particular could benefit from the use of a cream containing camomile. But so should people who have eczema. Ask at your health shop.

STIES: The first time I got one of these, I honestly thought a pig was coming to live in it! It was so big. If only I'd known about camomile tea. And not just for drinking! If you have a sty, make a compress with the tea and place it on the eye. The healing antiseptic qualities should do the trick.

STRESS: A lot of stress is down to the way we live. Camomile is very good for helping us unwind. If I'm facing a stressful situation, I drink a cup of camomile tea. The taste can sometime be a little toothpastey, but the end results are worth it because I feel much more relaxed dealing with things.

GINGIVITIS: Did I mention toothpaste? Camomile can treat gingivitis. It also makes a very good mouthwash because of its antiseptic qualities. If you suffer from gingivitis, then make a cup of camomile tea to use as a mouthwash after every meal.

ULCERS: Because camomile is such an aid to digestion, drinking camomile tea can help with stomach ulcers. This is because it possesses anti-inflammatory properties and soothes the stomach generally. If you're a sufferer, then taking a cup at bedtime could be beneficial.

AVAILABILITY: Camomile comes as a tea or a tincture. Most supermarkets stock the former and even offer mixes with other fruits and herbs.

A WORD OF CAUTION: If you suffer from hayfever, I'm sorry but you will have to use something else. Camomile is a member of the ragwort family and can irritate this condition. Also, if you experience any itching, discontinue use. Otherwise, camomile is a remedy you should keep handy in your cupboard.

INTERESTING FACT: The Victorians recommended camomile flowers for restoring tired or greying fair hair to its natural colour. After shampooing, they suggested pouring boiling water on camomile flowers, covering for fifteen minutes, straining, then pouring over the hair.

Carrots

Carrots are one of those vegetables we all take for granted. A rich source of beta-carotene (see page 133), studies have proven that carrots can help reduce the risk of cardiovascular disease and certain cancers. Instead of an apple a day, it's a carrot a day we need to munch. I'm only kidding about the apple, but seriously, eating a carrot a day could seriously improve our general health.

ANGINA: It's well known that vegetarians have a lower incidence of heart disease. This is partly because certain vegetables are full of calcium in addition to being generally less fatty. Some herbalists recommend juicing carrots with parsley, fennel, parsnips and water, and drinking the result in order to keep the heart healthy. If you don't fancy that, try our heart soup. The recipe's on pages 259–60.

DIARRHOEA: Carrots can be used to treat infant diarrhoea. Cook and cut or mash accordingly. When cooked, a small plate of carrots can soothe the digestive system and provide nutrients that can be lost during an attack. If the diarrhoea is serious or bloodstained, however, consult a doctor. Don't give your child too much. Make sure that what you are giving them is in tune with the amounts they are already eating.

SKIN PROBLEMS: Some herbalists recommend juicing carrots to put on minor skin conditions.

LIVER: Carrots can help detoxify the liver.

WRINKLES: Because carrots are high in vitamin A, they can help keep the skin moist and therefore help prevent wrinkles forming. Carrot oil makes a good face-mask. It can also be used as an effective sunscreen – thus doing two jobs at the same time. Certain sun oils do contain carrot oil. Have a good look for them next time you're in a chemist's or purchasing sun tan oil.

AVAILABILITY: Carrots are easy to buy, if you don't grow your own and they're also easy to eat. As well as serving them with a main course, you can eat carrot sticks and, of course, there's always soup. Carrot and coriander, made with orange juice, carrots, stock and coriander, is delicious, so is lentil, and what about our special healthy heart soup. You'll find it in the recipe section (page 159).

INTERESTING FACT: Carrots improved the vision of the Second World War fighter pilots, so it might do wonders for yours.

Celery

Celery contains a chemical that dilates the blood vessels generally, thus making it useful in helping sufferers of circulatory, heart and blood pressure problems. Again, I'm not saying it cures them, just that it makes sense to include it in your diet if you're a sufferer or worried about developing these conditions. It's a rather spicy vegetable to eat on its own, something of an acquired taste. If you don't like it, you can always try adding it to other vegetables, in a pasta dish, your favourite soup, whatever, so long as you are getting the benefits. And there should be benefits, especially if you suffer from the following.

ANGINA: Eating more vegetables generally can help improve this condition. Celery is particularly helpful because of its dilatory qualities. Try taking a portion each day combined with carrot.

GOUT: As well as improving circulation, celery helps the body get rid of uric acid which causes gout. You can try eating celery every day, or asking at your health shop for an extract containing celery in tablet form. Hopefully this will reduce the amount and severity of attacks by keeping the uric acid levels down.

GENERAL GOOD HEALTH: Eating celery regularly can help to provide the body with more energy. By keeping toxins down and improving circulation generally, you are keeping yourself in better shape. Celery has also been known to lower high blood pressure.

AVAILABILITY: Celery is easily obtainable and if you don't like it you can ask at your health shop for tablets containing celery extracts. If you're on a diet, the experts say that chewing a stick of celery will lessen your appetite. Why can't chocolate?

A WORD OF CAUTION: I personally don't know of anyone who has suffered ill effects from eating celery.

INTERESTING FACT: The Chinese have used celery for thousands of years to treat high blood pressure and vertigo.

Chiropractic

WHAT IS IT? While this therapy has been around a long time, modern chiropractic was founded in America in 1895. Apparently that's when one Mr Palmer – D.D. to his friends – restored the hearing of a man who had been deaf for 17 years, simply by adjusting one of his vertebrae. Manipulation of the spine was, he believed, the key to many bone, muscle and joint problems. Soon D.D. had set up his own school, and today chiropractic is one of the best-known alternative therapies going in America, although it's catching on elsewhere fast, too.

HOW DOES IT WORK? Obviously there are no prizes for guessing that it works by correcting any misalignment of the spine, neck or other problem areas. That's only part of it, however. Because it aims to restore the inner balance in your body, it also looks at your general health and makes sure the nervous system is flowing properly. Some chiropractors also look at diets and offer nutritional advice. Although a treatment might sound painful, very little force is used.

WHAT DOES IT HELP IN PARTICULAR? Although chiropractic is very good for relieving lower back pain, it also helps sore necks, joints and legs, migraine, muscle spasms, numbness and tingling in the nerves.

HOW LONG SHOULD A COURSE OF TREATMENT LAST? Like many other therapies, this depends on the condition. Usually the first visit takes an hour, while subsequent sessions take less – often as little as ten minutes. Some people find that one session is all they need. Others need two or three visits a week over a few weeks.

HOW DO I GO ABOUT GETTING THIS TREATMENT? Ask at your doctor's or health shop for the address of a local practitioner.

A WORD OF CAUTION: Always make sure your condition has been properly diagnosed before you embark on this therapy. If you have arthritis, sciatica or osteoporosis, then you must check with your doctor first. When you think about what is involved with chiropractic therapy, these conditions could easily be made worse, then you'll just be in more pain than ever and blaming the therapist. Or worse still, me! And that wouldn't do at all, now would it? Because chiropractic therapy involves a 'laying on of hands', choose a practitioner you feel comfortable with.

INTERESTING FACTS: Spinal manipulation has been around for thousands of years. Records of it go back to ancient China. The word itself derives from Greece.

Chitosan

As a highly experienced (and more often than not failed) dieter, I simply worship chitosan. Its dietary fibre is a great filler-upper, which is just what the dieter needs. Okay, it may not be chocolate, more's the pity, but it does the trick and very much tricks us into thinking we have just had a huge plateful!

Although this is purely my own theory (and that of all my, shall we say, less than svelte pals) chitosan fibre, combined with vitamin C, has reduced our appetites substantially, thus reducing the amount we eat. This should by no means be taken as read, however, as chitosan has no known side effects – it isn't actually a nutrient at all and therefore can cause no deficiency of any kind. And, as vitamin C is not absorbable, it will not cause any harm. It will simply, to put it mildly, go in one end and make its way south, where it subsequently comes out the other end! No harmful side effects there and, moreover, perhaps a better chance of losing unwanted weight!

On a more serious note, chitosan has a few good qualities and benefits in its own right. Found and extracted from the shells of shrimp and crabs, it remains a supplement suited to some preventions.

CHOLESTEROL: Some studies have shown that the consumption of chitosan may lower blood cholesterol while also raising levels of HDL (high density lipoprotein), more commonly known as essential cholesterol.

HIGH BLOOD PRESSURE: Although by no means yet fact, early studies show that chitosan, while not necessarily lowering blood pressure as such, seems to prevent any worrying rise in blood pressure.

KIDNEYS: Again, some early studies show that improved kidney functions occur in those using chitosan.

SOFTLY, SOFTLY: I've named this heading so, because, a very small study shows that chitosan may, and I reiterate *may*, help prevent intestinal disease such as colon cancer.

A WORD OF CAUTION: Overall I would have to recommend – despite my own, very layman-type beliefs – that chitosan is treated with great respect. I sense it is one of the newer supplements and that research has not yet been thorough enough nor extensive enough to prove anything either way. One huge and very clear warning, which I came across repeatedly whilst studying chitosan, is that those with any kind of malabsorption disorder, should steer well clear of chitosan, as should children and pregnant women.

INTERESTING FACTS: A few years ago, during a visit to friends in London, an article was read out to me about this apparently new supplement. The article clearly claimed how beneficial it was for those dieting and, as a result, I immediately purchased huge quantities of chitosan fibre supplements!

Cinnamon

If you're surprised at what such a sweet little spice is doing here, well I'll tell you. It's because it heals so many things – fever, heartburn and nausea, to mention but a few – and has a history going back 4,000 years. Can't be bad! And you just thought it was nice in cakes and buns! Well, it is too. That's actually one of my favourite uses. But there are others, and here are some.

FEVER: Historically, cinnamon has an anti-fever reputation. If you have a fever, try a cup of cinnamon tea to bring the temperature down.

HEARTBURN: If you're a regular sufferer, then try sprinkling even a little cinnamon on some of your food, eating food with cinnamon in it, or drinking cinnamon tea. Cinnamon aids digestion generally, you'll find, eliminating the acids and gases that cause problems.

NAUSEA: Some of the chemicals in cinnamon are called catechins, which help relieve nausea. So if you feel you are going to be sick, try taking cinnamon tea, or a drop of tincture to relieve the symptoms. One drop only please. (See page 153.)

YEAST INFECTION: Oral candida can be improved with cinnamon oil. It contains antibacterial qualities, which may also help with mouth ulcers.

ERECTION PROBLEMS: Because cinnamon generates the blood flow you might even find it helps with this!

AVAILABILITY: Cinnamon is available in sticks, powdered, as a tincture or as an oil and is very easily come by. Oils and tincture are available from your health shop. Remember not to take the oil unless it recommends you to do so on the label. Cinnamon oil is strong. Powdered cinnamon is easy to find in most supermarkets and a tea can be made by pouring a cup of boiling water on two grams, allowing it to cool, then drinking.

A WORD OF CAUTION: Cinnamon is not recommended for pregnant women. Some people develop dermatitis after using cinnamon. If you're one, discontinue use. The concentrated oil is more of a problem in this respect.

INTERESTING FACT: Cinnamon may be the oldest herbal medicine. The Chinese used it 4,000 years ago. Other cultures used it to treat arthritis and various menstrual disorders.

Cloves

Traditionally, cloves have been recognised as antiseptics and pain relievers. I'm sure we can all remember our mothers reaching into the medicine cabinet for Oil of Cloves when we had toothache or earache as a child. Indeed there was a time when no self-respecting first aid kit was without this. Of course, in some instances, you have to dilute and warm the oil first, as I soon found out when I poured it in someone's ears once. So do be careful. Use it properly. And also, remember not to take the oil, it's for external use only.

ALTITUDE SICKNESS: Clove oil contains a compound that helps thin the blood. The oil can't be taken, but if you steep some cloves (not the oil) in a cup of boiling water you should get the same effect. You could also try adding some cinnamon to taste – something that makes it sound a bit like a mulled wine – then, when the liquid has cooled, drink the result. Of course you can't go looking for cloves and cinnamon once you're halfway up the mountain. The thing to do is have the tea before you start. Or brew it up and take it with you.

TOOTHACHE: Because clove oil has an anaesthetic effect, it's very good for toothache, although of course any persistent toothache should be checked by a dentist. Most people suffering toothache do go to a dentist anyway. This is a helpful stopgap remedy, however. Just place a few drops of the oil on the tooth when needed.

CUTS AND SCRAPES: Sprinkling powdered cloves on a cut can stop it from becoming infected.

A WORD OF CAUTION: As I've already said never take the oil. It's for external use only. If you want to dilute it, add a little vegetable oil and if you do heat it, make sure it has cooled to a warm temperature before pouring it on the skin. Otherwise, clove oil is safe to use, as are powdered cloves.

INTERESTING FACT: I like this one. When people of ancient Asian cultures wanted to see the king, they had to chew cloves first. This was so they wouldn't offend the royal person with any niffy odours.

Comfrey

Comfrey is another herb that has been used for thousands of years. It has, however, fallen out of favour because it contains potentially dangerous compounds, toxic to the liver in particular. However, there is no harm in applying comfrey to the skin and, used properly, it has many healing qualities.

BRUISES: Comfrey contains anti-inflammatory compounds that promote healing as well as reducing the inflammation. It is especially helpful for bruises and skin discoloration. You can simmer comfrey root in water for ten minutes, soak a piece of cloth in the liquid, then apply it to the skin. If you don't fancy doing that, ask at your health shop for a cream containing comfrey.

STRAINS: A strained wrist or ankle can be treated in the same way as a bruise (see above).

DANDRUFF: Either ask at your health shop for a shampoo containing comfrey or add a few drops of tincture to your normal shampoo. Comfrey has properties that help clear dandruff and heal the scalp so that it doesn't flake.

SORES: If you follow the procedure for treating bruises, you might find that external ulcers and sores that won't heal can be helped by applying a poultice of comfrey leaf or root in the first instance. Then you can use a cream to complete the healing and mend scarring.

AVAILABILITY: You can buy tincture and cream containing comfrey from your health shop, or grow your own and pick the leaves and use the root to make compresses and poultices.

A WORD OF CAUTION: Well I've a big one actually. Comfrey does contain some very dangerous compounds, so I would not suggest taking it internally, unless it is being sold for that use. Some people have drunk comfrey tea for years with absolutely no ill effects, but we're not all the same and others have developed problems with their livers. Pregnant and breast-feeding women are advised against using comfrey, certainly internally. Externally, as a healing agent, it appears safe.

INTERESTING FACT: The ancient Greeks used comfrey to heal wounds. One of my readers wrote telling me she uses comfrey as a poultice on her thrombosis.

Cranberry

A relative of the blueberry, cranberries are grown across Europe and America and are often found in marshy ground. Small and red in appearance they have a bitter taste, which makes them unpleasant to eat on their own. However, there are a variety of ways of taking cranberries – including putting the juice on food as a sauce – and they do such good. Recent studies show that drinking a glass of cranberry juice every day is very beneficial to good health. Moreover, cranberry juice is very readily available in a way that it wasn't a few years ago. So get drinking. Mixed with other juices it is also very pleasant as a non-alcoholic alternative to red wine for people who don't drink alcohol.

You can make a good non-alcoholic alternative to red wine by mixing it half-and-half with blackcurrant juice, a cup of water and a cup of orange. You can even make a very good alcoholic punch by mixing it with red wine and raspberry. Then there's cranberry pie and cranberry fudge. Absolutely delicious, both of them, although the latter does pile on the calories a little! Our recipes for both are at the back of the book in appendix 1. Happy eating!

BLADDER INFECTIONS: Cranberry and blueberry both contain arbutin, a compound that is both an antibiotic and a diuretic. So drinking juice regularly is not only boosting good health in general but may help cut down on this kind of infection, particularly if you are a frequent sufferer. Arbutin helps by flushing the bacteria out from the bladder wall.

FEVER: As cranberry has an anti-fever reputation, taking cranberry juice when you have a cold or flu may help reduce your fever. You can warm it a little by heating it in a pot and even add some blackcurrant juice to sweeten it and a little sprinkling of cinnamon (or put a cinnamon stick in it) to give it that 'ye olde fashioned cold remedy' taste. With a little dash of freshly squeezed orange and a slice of lemon it's perfect and a great way of treating a cold.

ASTHMA: While not so potent as some other herbs or vegetables, cranberry contains some anti-asthmatic substances. So perhaps the above recipe might help sufferers.

CANDIDA: Arbutin can also help with candida. So if you're troubled, drink lots of juice regularly, or put cranberry sauce on your food.

A WORD OF CAUTION: As always, consult your GP if any particular problem isn't relieved after a short period of time.

INTERESTING FACT: The best cranberries come from the mountains of Virginia. Cranberries were, once upon a time, used as poultices for the treatment of scurvy (a vitamin C deficiency).

Craniosacral therapy

WHAT IS IT? Although it sounds as if it's not for the faint hearted and a bit gory to boot, craniosacral therapy is actually a gentle form of manipulation. Therapists work with the soft tissue and bones of the head, the spine and the membranes that surround these bones. It's done with such a light touch, most people are hardly aware of it taking place.

HOW DOES IT WORK? Well, therapists think that it's the movement of spinal fluid through the nervous system that keeps us healthy. If the system is blocked, perhaps by injury, then health problems result. Gentle manipulation, however, helps get things back to normal so to speak, restoring the body's natural balance.

WHAT DOES IT HELP IN PARTICULAR? Craniosacral therapy has been shown to reduce stress, improve the quality of sleep and generally boost well being. It is also thought it can help headaches, dizziness, tinnitus and sinusitis.

HOW LONG SHOULD A COURSE OF TREATMENT LAST? A typical session lasts from 20 minutes to an hour and the number of sessions depends on the problem. Some can be solved in one session. Others require several weekly sessions.

HOW DO I GO ABOUT GETTING THIS TREATMENT? Ask at your health centre or health shop for a properly trained practitioner.

A WORD OF CAUTION: If you have ever had that headache to end all headaches (i.e. a brain haemorrhage or aneurysm) then this treatment might not be for you. See your doctor first. Craniosacral therapy is also not for life-threatening problems such as cancer or heart disease. Also, remember to choose your practitioner with care and make sure they are properly qualified, otherwise you could end up with more problems than you had previously. This therapy has recently become popular for young children. I can certainly think of one little colicky baby who benefited! You must, however, take special care to ensure that your child is only treated by a properly trained practitioner if you are considering this treatment.

INTERESTING FACT: Craniosacral therapy is one of the babies when it comes to alternative medicine. It was only discovered in the 1930s by an American osteopath.

Damiana

Despite research showing that this amazing herbal remedy contains testosterone, a male hormone, I always equate it with women and women's problems. I have my favourites, as we all do, but damiana has to stand out – like echinacea, which I lovingly term as 'my male remedy' – as the 'female remedy'.

Damiana is a powerful remedy and one that can be used for a diverse number of ailments such as depression, anxiety, headaches and bed wetting. It is found in Mexico, where its dry, aromatic leaves are used in capsule form, tincture or teas. It can also be used as an inhalant once the tea itself is brewed.

LOWERING BLOOD SUGAR: Not only is damiana thought to have antibacterial qualities but it also appears to have abilities in lowering blood sugar levels for those suffering from diabetes.

NERVOUS SYSTEM: It is believed that damiana strengthens the nervous system, thus meaning it can help relieve problems caused by depression. I have found it to be a great, all-round 'pick me up' and have recommended it a great many times to clients. I have yet to hear it has failed in its quest to suppress depression.

POST-NATAL DEPRESSION: Not only is damiana good for strengthening the central nervous system but it also seems able to tackle the hormonal system. This means it can be used for PMT, menopause and postnatal depression.

CONSTIPATION: I did say it was diverse – well how much more diverse can something be? Damiana also has compounds that have a laxative effect. It can also be used for urinary infection, so you are just about covered for many ailments if you use damiana regularly.

HEADACHE: A pleasant way to take damiana is as a tea. By steeping one teaspoonful of the dried herb in a cup of hot water and drinking three times a day, you can inhale its aroma and relieve headaches, especially tension headaches.

A WORD OF CAUTION: The only one I've come across is that it should, like most other edibles, be used in moderation. As always, follow the manufacturer's guidelines.

INTERESTING FACTS: Damiana is thought to be of benefit to the man's sexual system. In fact, damiana is believed to be an aphrodisiac.

Dandelion

More often than not the dandelion is regarded as an out-and-out pest, a hard-to-remove weed that grows at random, usually in the middle of our prized lawns or window boxes. It is hard to believe, therefore, that in Europe this plant is so prized, it is actually grown commercially, and there was even a time in Britain when no decent herb garden would have been without a sizeable clump.

Dandelion is sometimes called by another name, all to do with bed-wetting, which being polite I won't repeat here, but suffice to say it is appropriate. The leaves and roots have diuretic qualities, meaning they help to flush excess water from the body. While this cannot cure a bladder infection, it can flush the urine out, thus getting rid of some of the bacteria that causes these infections.

For many centuries, too, the root heads have been used to treat conditions of the liver, such as jaundice, but the flowers too contain lecithin, a nutrient that has been proven to be useful in various liver ailments. In addition to the roots, the flower has a high concentration of vitamins A and B, both helpful in the treatment of liver conditions.

Lecithin itself has been shown to improve the memory in laboratory mice. While this does not necessarily prove that dandelion is good for our memory, it is certainly worth considering if you are prone to forgetting things or perhaps want to sharpen your memory for exams.

CONSTIPATION: Dandelion in tea form is good for this irritating and inconvenient condition. With its high concentration of vitamins, one cup three times a day should do the trick.

ANAEMIA: Dandelion can strengthen the blood. Simply take one teaspoon of fresh juice, or tincture with water, twice a day.

MASTITIS: The Chinese boil a teaspoonful of minced dandelion root in two cups of water to make a compress to treat mastitis.

TONSILLITIS: As if this isn't enough, using the same recipe but boiled down until only half the liquid remains, makes a syrup that is great for tonsillitis.

A WORD OF CAUTION: Reading all this might well be enough to send you dancing out to the garden to pluck up all these dandelions that have been littering your paths for ages, cast them into a pot and start curing everything that's ever been wrong with you. Indeed, some herbalists do suggest boiling, or steaming, the plant like spinach in order to eat or drink the resulting concoction. However, just think about all the fertilisers, pesticides, etc., you may have sprayed the garden with – not to mention the odd passing cat or dog – and it's enough to make you change your mind. Unless you can be really sure, you should pay a visit to your local health food store, where you can buy various products containing dandelion, such as root tea, juice, or tincture. Also, don't take dandelion if you have persistent constipation, as this may be a sign of obstruction, or if you are pregnant or breast-feeding.

INTERESTING FACTS: Employees of the Hudson Bay Company, which was founded in 1670, received regular shipments of dandelion roots to supplement their meat-laden diet. The name means lion's tooth – dente de lion. Take a look at its pointy leaves to see why. In olden days, girls used to pick the ripe seed heads and blow them away. The number of puffs taken was supposed to tell how many years it would be till they were married.

Dill

With the current preference for shortening names, dill sounds a bit like a soap star to me. It is, however, a particularly useful herb, especially in the treatment of stomach conditions – all those nasty things like wind and bad breath. So, if you're system isn't all it should be in that respect, i.e. if you suffer from general heartburn, upsets and poor digestion, this one's for you. I would certainly recommend it for the following conditions.

COLIC: Colic can vary from mild to extremely painful and be a real bugbear, especially if you're out. I didn't say pain there, we already know it's that! Because dill aids digestion generally, it can help prevent attacks. See below for how to make a tea, if you've got a dose. Otherwise, just adding it to your food can help cut down on the number you suffer. If this is a problem for you, consider it.

WIND: If you suffer regularly from this not very nice condition, a number of herbs can help. (See Flatulence, pages 50–1.) One of them is dill, which actually contains compounds that relieve it. When you're cooking, try adding a sprinkling to your food. It does make for better digestion generally.

HEARTBURN: If you're a sufferer, then try crushing a teaspoonful of seeds in a cup and adding boiling water, then, when it's cool, sipping it. Alternatively, it would do no harm to use a little in your cooking so that your body is absorbing it as you eat, making sure of good digestion afterwards.

A WORD OF CAUTION: Do not take dill if you are pregnant, as this can cause problems.

INTERESTING FACT: Dill has been used for thousands of years for the treatment of heartburn.

Echinacea

The common name for the very difficult and often wrongly pronounced echinacea ('eck-in-ay-sha') is Purple Coneflower. Echinacea is native to North America and is gathered from the wild. It is said that little of the flower is wasted and that, in fact, most of it is used: flowers, roots, stems and leaves.

I call this 'the man's remedy' although it is used for a great many other purposes. This is strictly my own personal opinion and I derive such a conclusion, I guess, from the fact that it is mainly to the male of the species that I recommend this herb.

On the whole, echinacea is one of my most used, most recommended and overall favourite of all herbs, vitamins and the like. This is purely down to its amazingly versatile curing ability.

Echinacea can be beneficial to those with sore throats, infections, bronchitis, gingivitis, cold sores and mouth ulcers to name but a few. It is, however, best summarised as a good old immune booster.

COMMON COLD: If taken early enough, particularly on the onset of a cold or sore throat, this herb can in fact deter and quite frankly stop dead in its tracks any cold, virus and even flu. It most definitely has been proven to reduce susceptibility to these ailments. It is best advised to use echinacea regularly, thus preventing even an onset of colds and the like. If you already have a full-blown cold, sore throat, etc., then using this herb can both lessen its severity, as well as hasten your recovery.

CANCER (as you will see, I am attempting to steer clear of such sinister and often fatal illnesses): As this herb has renowned immunity strengthening qualities, it has been noted that using it can indeed benefit the immune system during cancer treatments, thus possibly prolonging life. Some proof has emerged to substantiate this claim.

CHRONIC FATIGUE SYNDROME: This somewhat controversial, although, in my opinion, very real syndrome can be reduced or even thwarted by the use of echinacea. This is due once again to its amazing capacity to give the immune system a huge boost.

SKIN: Burns, mouth ulcers, cuts, grazes, herpes (including genital), shingles and the like can all be healed at a faster rate by using echinacea. This is down to the fact that this amazing herb is also a wonderful and natural antibiotic.

A WORD OF CAUTION: Although I clearly adore this herb, it should not be used as an alternative to conventional antibiotics but rather as well as. It should not be used for those suffering from Lupus or any one of the autoimmune disorders.

INTERESTING FACTS: I could write an entire book alone on the benefits of this herb. Echinacea comes in many forms – e.g.

tablets, dried herbs, capsules, lozenges, tincture and liquid (liquid being a bit too bitter for my liking!).

Elderberry

Every time I hear the word elderberry, I always think of the Joseph Kesselring play *Arsenic and Old Lace* and the two old ladies saying, 'It's elderberry wine,' as they hand over their murderous potion to their unsuspecting lodgers. To be fair, it was really the arsenic content that accounted for the bodies in the cellar. Elderberry itself has many uses, particularly in the treatment of colds and flu and is fairly simple to take. Much simpler than the 'gentleman lodgers' found it. Personally, I rather like it – and elderberry wine, of course!

COUGH: Elderberry can be very useful for treating colds, but sometimes a cough can linger for weeks after and be troublesome. Drinking elderberry tea could help, or you could try adding a few drops of tincture to another herbal tea. Take two or three cups a day, till the cough has gone. A client of mine did this recently and enjoyed it so much, she added it to her shopping list. As for the cough, it disappeared, so perhaps there's something in it!

TONSILLITIS: Elderberry juice features prominently as a traditional treatment for tonsillitis. Ask at your health store if you are a regular sufferer. You might find that incorporating it into your diet helps in the long run.

IMMUNE SYSTEM: Because of its centuries' old reputation as a healer, elderberry can help boost your immune system generally.

FLU: Flu is an absolute misery and difficult to treat, let's be honest. There are no magic cures. However, Israeli scientists discovered that a drug made from elderberries significantly helped flu victims recover. Muscle aches were relieved and fever reduced. Moreover, sufferers recovered far quicker. Elderberry tea or juice could help. You can even try making up a hot drink with cranberry and raspberry juice (see Cranberry, page 155). Don't wait till you have the symptoms, keep some tea bags or juice handy in you medicine cupboard, with some zinc lozenges, so if flu strikes you won't be caught out.

AVAILABILITY: Elderberry comes as a juice, in tea form, as a jam, or a wine. You might even have a tree in your garden and can pick the berries yourself, boiling them into a syrup that can be added to tea. It is unlikely to do you any harm unless there are any strange old ladies with murderous intentions nearby.

A WORD OF CAUTION: Fresh elderberry can produce allergies when handled. Try to avoid allowing children to handle the freshly grown ones. Otherwise, cooked, powdered, tea bags, etc. are safe.

INTERESTING FACTS: According to German folklore, the hat must be doffed when you pass an elder tree. In Denmark too, the tree was said to be under the protection of the earth mother and its flowers could not be gathered without her permission. The cross of Christ was said to be made from elder wood. It was also a common medieval tradition that Judas hanged himself on an elder tree. It was thought unlucky to place a baby in an elder-wood cradle.

Eucalyptus

Originally used by the Australian aborigines for soothing painful joints and healing cuts, the leaves and oil of the eucalyptus tree were also used to fight infection and treat wounds in the pre-antibiotic era.

The tree itself originates from Australia, whose inhabitants take great pride in classing it 'their find'. However, eucalyptus trees are now grown worldwide.

COUGHS AND COLDS: When inhaled, eucalyptus oil works as an expectorant, loosening sticky mucus, so that victims of colds, flu, asthma, sinusitis and croup can breath more easily. Because it opens the tube between the middle ear and the throat, earache, which is often linked to some of the above illnesses, can also be relieved by the inhalation of eucalyptus oil.

TO INHALE: Add one or two drops of eucalyptus oil to a pan of water and boil. Drape a towel over your head and lean towards the pan and inhale deeply through the nostrils. Repeat twice daily, more frequently for earaches. Protect yourself from the oil's fumes by keeping your eyes shut when inhaling. If you don't fancy inhaling, eucalyptus tea is readily available from good health stores. Drink two cups per day until symptoms subside.

FOR MUSCLE ACHES AND PAINS: Rub several drops of commercially diluted oil into the affected area or soak in a herbal bath made by running the bath water through a handful of leaves, wrapped in cheesecloth.

GUM DISEASE: Can also be fought by massaging several drops of commercially diluted eucalyptus oil onto the affected area. This reduces plaque. Look in your local supermarket for toothpastes containing eucalyptus oil.

A WORD OF CAUTION: Eucalyptus oil products should never be applied to the face of an infant or small child because it can cause severe asthma-like reactions. It should not be used by pregnant women. When used as recommended, and with care, eucalyptus products are safe, but swallowing even a small amount of undiluted oil can cause serious reactions, including a drop in blood pressure and temperature. So this is one remedy that must always be treated with care.

INTERESTING FACTS: Historically, chewing eucalyptus roots provided the aborigines with water in the otherwise very dry outback. Eucalyptus oil was used by some surgeons as a sterilising agent for their surgical instruments.

Evening primrose oil

Evening primrose oil is one of those wonderful remedies that would probably need a whole book devoted to it. Not quite, but just about! And unfortunately it isn't possible to take a look at all of its properties here. With research ongoing into many conditions and illnesses, it may be that evening primrose oil has a role to play in reducing tumours. One of its main properties is an acid that acts as a blood thinner and anti-inflammatory and although many people have adequate levels of this substance others do not. So it may be that if you suffer from the following, you don't, and a capsule containing evening primrose oil would help.

DRY MOUTH: If you're a sufferer, you can soothe away this problem by taking evening primrose capsules regularly. They help stimulate salivation and equally lessen that prickly throat sensation that goes with it.

HEADACHE: If you suffer regularly from headaches, then taking evening primrose oil can help. However, it might not keep them away entirely. You would also have to take the capsules on a daily basis, sometimes several times a day, depending on the dosage, for them to be effective. But they are certainly worth a shot.

PRE-MENSTRUAL TENSION: I recommended evening primrose oil for one client who was suffering very badly from this condition and she found that it definitely helped reduce the bloated feeling and anxiety and made her feel so much better that she's been taking it since. I didn't just need her to tell me. There are several studies that say just the same thing. If you suffer from this and are unbearable at that time of the month and find life unbearable, then try taking the capsules prior to and during your period. You can buy them at your supermarket or health shop.

MENSTRUAL CRAMPS: You might also find that another benefit of taking the oil is to reduce cramps and generally regulate the flow. Take as directed.

ECZEMA: Evening primrose is approved in Britain for treating eczema. If it's never been suggested to you, then I'm doing so now. Take as directed.

SCABIES: Skin mite infestation is the cause of this condition, which is often common amongst children these days rather than adults. Since evening primrose oil is useful for eczema, you can probably give it a try for this, being careful to follow the dosage instructions.

SKIN PROBLEMS: Other skin problems, such as dermatitis, might improve with regular daily intakes of this oil. If you're a sufferer and you don't know why, then it might be because of a deficiency (see page 166), in which case this is definitely worth checking out. If your problem disappears, then that's what it's been.

RHEUMATOID ARTHRITIS: Some studies have shown that sufferers improved when taking evening primrose oil. I can only say that if all else has failed, or you think you're at risk, then please give this a try. Evening primrose oil does possess anti-inflammatory properties, which might give you some relief from your symptoms.

AVAILABILITY: Evening primrose oil comes in capsule or tablet form, available from supermarkets and health shops.

A WORD OF CAUTION: None that I know of, but remember to follow the instructions.

INTERESTING FACT: For hundreds of years Native Americans have chewed the seeds to relieve menstrual problems. Being the hypochondriac that I am, I take evening primrose oil daily – just in case!

Fennel

So here's another one I bet you thought was just a troublesome old weed! Historically, however, the seeds have been used to cure many medical conditions. It's also interesting to note that these conditions vary from culture to culture. Fennel contains many constituents, so perhaps that explains it. It can also be used as a cooking spice, especially with fish. One legend has it that fennel may have bestowed immortality. Obviously I can't swear to that but I can say that it can improve your health!

HEARTBURN: Fennel comes into its own when it comes to dealing with stomach ailments like heartburn, indigestion and wind. The seeds contain a constituent that stops painful spasms. Whole seeds can be chewed, as people in many cultures do after a meal, or crushed to make a tea by pouring boiling water over. It's one teaspoon of crushed seeds to a cup, by the way. If you don't fancy this, ask at your health shop for a tincture, tablets, or any drink containing fennel and take according to the instructions.

ASTHMA: One of the compounds in fennel makes it useful as an expectorant. You could try taking it as a tea each day to see if it helps with this condition.

COLIC: Fennel can be used to help infant sufferers of colic. If you have a tricky baby in this respect, ask at your health shop for a soothing fennel drink.

LOSS OF LIBIDO: Some of the compounds in fennel are similar to oestrogen. You might find, therefore, that a cup of fennel tea twice a day helps get things going in this department!

BREAST-FEEDING: Again, fennel was used in America to stimulate milk flow. Not only this but it was used elsewhere for centuries to do the same. If you have a problem it might be worth trying a cup of fennel tea two times a day to get things going. Since fennel can help infant colic, it shouldn't be a problem for the baby either.

BLADDER INFECTIONS: Some studies have recently shown that fennel can act as a diuretic. It's certainly worth a shot if you suffer on a regular basis. A fennel tea or drink would be best. Ask at your health shop or make your own from the seeds. Remember to take according to the instructions.

A WORD OF CAUTION: In some rare instances, fennel can cause an allergic reaction of the skin and respiratory tract. Certain cancer sufferers, too, should not take fennel. Therefore, please consult your doctor, if you're thinking about it. While fennel tea made from fennel seeds is safe to drink, please don't take fennel oil. If you are pregnant, it can cause a miscarriage. It is also highly toxic.

INTERESTING FACT: Fennel is actually cultivated in many parts of Asia.

Feverfew

Grown widely right across Europe, feverfew is used for many ailments but is most famous for its ability to ease the agony of migraine. In general, however, it is widely used for its overall pain-killing abilities. For centuries healers relied on this remarkable plant and its aroma to treat headaches, stomach upsets, menstrual cramps, fever (obviously!) and even repel insects, purify the air and prevent disease – a tall order indeed. But its qualities were largely forgotten until the 1970s. Its powers are attributed to the presence of the chemical parthenolide and, without being too technical, it's worth stressing that unless the form you buy has this magic word on the label, it won't do a lot of good. Certainly not the good that's intended. Many of its other properties are similar to aspirin so it's wise to avoid using one in combination with the other.

MIGRAINES: Exactly how feverfew helps migraines is unclear. When taken preventively it can lessen the intensity of one, however, as well as the nausea so often associated with it. To be properly effective it has to be taken regularly for several weeks in tablet form, but don't expect miracle results on a one-off basis or when the migraine has taken hold. Feverfew will not help then, however much you may want it to.

MENSTRUAL CRAMPS: These occur because the lining of the uterus produces too much prostaglandin, a hormone that causes inflammation. Feverfew has known properties that reduce inflammation. Try taking feverfew capsules, two times on the day before you think your period is due and again for a day or two after, and see what the results are.

ARTHRITIS: At its most acute, feverfew has been known to reduce swelling and so ease the pain associated with this often crippling disease.

AVAILABILITY: Feverfew comes in many forms: tablet, fresh herb, tea, capsule and as a tincture. On the whole it has a bitter taste, however, and most users therefore prefer to take it as a tablet.

A WORD OF CAUTION: Due to its many properties similar to aspirin, it is advisable not to take other drugs containing aspirin along with feverfew. Aspirin, as I think we all know by now, can irritate the stomach, so caution is advised. Pregnant and lactating women are advised against the use of feverfew, as are children under the age of two.

INTERESTING FACTS: Chewing feverfew leaves can be beneficial, too, for the lessening of pain. However, it has been documented that doing so can cause mouth ulcers in some people – a contradictory statement considering it is often used to reduce swelling.

Figs

Figs are known to possess, in an unusually high degree, two important food qualities: a definite laxative effect and a high excess of alkalinity of ash. In some cultures, the leaves and bark of the fig tree, as well as the fruits themselves, are used in native folk medicines.

CONSTIPATION: Historically, figs have been used to treat this condition and are available from any chemist's counter in syrup form. Follow the instructions as regards dosage. If you are a regular sufferer, then try adding figs to your diet. I know one old lady who swears by fig rolls and eats one a day to keep her system regular. She's 87 by the way, and, apart from being a little forgetful, she's very healthy. If constipation persists, you should see a doctor, however, as this may be a sign of an obstruction, something figs certainly won't cure.

CORNS: Although the best way to treat corns is to stop them developing in the first place, that's easier said than done and hardly the kind of helpful advice you want here, if you've got one. If you have, cut open a fig and tape it over the area overnight. Don't laugh. Figs contain powerful enzymes that dissolve unwanted skin growths. In the morning, remove the fig and soak the foot in warm water. After an hour or so the corn should come off but you can rub it with a pumice stone to make sure.

WARTS: As with corns, warts can be treated with figs. It's all right, I'm not going to suggest taping one to your finger. You'd get some very odd looks doing that. Traditionally, herbalists recommended squeezing the figs to get the milk, then spreading it on the wart. You would, however, have to do this several times before seeing any affect.

AVAILABILITY: Figs are readily available dried or fresh, as a syrup or in biscuit form, all from supermarkets.

A WORD OF CAUTION: The chief element in dried figs is sugar, so it might not be advisable to eat them if you suffer from diabetes.

INTERESTING FACTS: When King Solomon developed boils, what did his physician prescribe? Figs of course. In Mediterranean countries the fig is so widely used it is called 'the poor man's food'. Buddha was said to have become endued with his divine powers whilst sitting under a sacred fig tree in Ceylon. The fig is revered as being sacred by Buddhists and Brahmans in India.

Fruit

These days it's easier to come by fruit than ever. Just check out your local supermarket for a start. And exotic fruits too. I think I would be here all day if I tried to get round them all. So what I will say is that all fresh fruit is good for you and if you can eat a piece or two each day, then it's helping keep your digestive system in good order, naturally, as well as giving you certain vitamins and minerals. Whatever fruit you choose is up to you of course. We all have different tastes. Below are some of the better known ones, which also have certain healing and preventative benefits.

APPLE: You know the saying about an apple, and I have to say I'm in agreement with it. I'm not saying it keeps the doctor away, but it does keep the body in good working order. In fact, it's one of these strange things that can be recommended for both constipation and diarrhoea! It's also good for freshening the breath after a meal, if you can't clean your teeth. Making a mash by simmering washed, sliced, but unpeeled, apples in a saucepan with a little water, can help a cold. Just simmer for an hour in a covered pan, strain, then drink. Adding a spoonful of honey should also help.

BANANA: Did you know that bananas are very good for gastro-intestinal problems? Traditionally, they were used to help soothe upset stomachs. If you suffer from stomach problems or want to keep your digestive health good, avoiding things like ulcers, then a banana a day would go a long way towards that.

GRAPES: Red grapes or red grape juice has compounds that help to lower cholesterol. So if you want to keep your heart fit, or are worried at all about heart disease, perhaps because it runs in your family, then eating or drinking some every day is a very good way of keeping this organ fit. Green and red grapes both contain anti-arthritic, anti-inflammatory compounds, making them good to take to help reduce your chances of getting this, as well as helping to reduce the pain if you are a sufferer. Grapes are also good for reducing wrinkles. Just put them in a liquidiser and mash. The grapes that is! Wouldn't it be wonderful to do the same with the wrinkles! Then apply the mash to your face for 20 minutes. Grape juice is also excellent for settling a gippy tummy, where the upset is caused by an allergic reaction to food or a drug. Just drink a glass of juice mixed with water.

LEMON: Lemons are rather too sour for my personal taste. The juice and rinds are, however, good for colds. The recipe is the juice of one lemon, one tablespoon of honey and one teaspoon of sage in a cup of boiling water for 15 minutes. Strain, then drink. Lemon juice in hot water makes a good gargle for a sore throat. Lemon juice is also good for wasp stings. Just dab it on. And speaking of insects, they don't like the smell, making it an ideal repellent if you squeeze some on your skin.

ORANGE: Oranges are a very good source of vitamin C and a glass of freshly squeezed orange juice is still one of the best and most natural remedies there is for constipation.

PEACH: The Chinese use peach leaves to help cure morning sickness. They make a tea by steeping them in hot water.

PEAR: Traditionally, pears were used to tempt the appetite of the sick, especially if the pears had been soaked in red wine and cooked in honey. It does sound nice, I must admit. Pears contain some good anti-viral compounds, too, which no doubt did the trick as well. If you want to give your immune system a real boost, then you can't go wrong with a pear a day.

PINEAPPLE: Fresh pineapples are excellent for several conditions. They contain a substance that reduces inflammation, something that makes them particularly useful for treating sport's injuries and tendinitis. Arthritis sufferers, too, might find it's worth including them in their diet along with grapes. While they might not cure the arthritis they can certainly help and so much of a condition and how you manage it can be down to what you eat. The same goes for gout sufferers. A glass of pineapple juice each day might help keep the condition under control. While sufferers from stomach ulcers, indigestion – heartburn might find that this is one dietary requirement that really does help. That's because they're full of digestive enzymes. Pineapples are also very good for skin care generally. Look for a cream or lotion containing them and smooth away wrinkles and spots. Or blend the skin and husk and apply to the face for ten minutes.

A WORD OF CAUTION: I can't think of any where fruit is concerned except to say that some people can have allergies to certain things. I have a friend who can't eat limes or anything with lime flavouring in it, for instance. So if you're allergic to something of course you shouldn't take it.

INTERESTING FACT: Apple juice was traditionally used to treat dandruff, and lemon juice to make hair shine.

Garlic

So here's one that not only keeps the vampires at bay but also – as you can see below – helps if they do bite you! Garlic has many uses, so many I think you should refer to the Glossary of Herbal Remedies (pages 289–96) for a fuller picture. For thousands of years it has been recognised as quite a powerful healer, although of course it does have its little drawbacks. Stinky breath for one. No wonder it kept back the vampires, and probably anyone else coming within a foot's breadth! Seriously, I like garlic as a food flavouring, that's why I ladle it in everything. But I know not everyone's like me. Garlic capsules are now widely available and, what's more, are often odourless, which is good news for those who don't like the smell. So get on the garlic. You could do a lot worse!

ALLERGIES: It seems that everywhere you turn these days, someone has an allergy to something. Garlic is one of those helpful herbs that helps stop inflammatory reactions. Start adding it to your cooking, or have the capsules handy if you find your nasal passages clog and you can't stop sneezing.

ALTITUDE SICKNESS: Climbers take note. Garlic contains substances that thin the blood and is a good preventative to altitude sickness. You could try taking some in your food before you climb.

ANGINA/HEART DISEASE: Garlic actually helps lower cholesterol and blood pressure, so is excellent if you suffer from heart disease.

COLDS AND FLU: Garlic has long been recognised as the herbal antibiotic. We all make jokes about the smell but it's precisely its aromatic compounds that go straight to the respiratory tract, making it ideal for treating most respiratory illnesses. Either get on the garlic and onion soup, if you've got a cold, or take capsules. Also, while you might not avoid colds entirely, you can stay a lot healthier generally by simply taking as much as you can in your food by way of garlic bread, salad dressings, or simply toss it in the rice, pasta or pizza topping.

BURNS: As well as having antiviral, antibiotic qualities, this remarkable plant is also antiseptic. It can be used to treat burns. Just mash some powder or fresh cloves to a paste and apply as a poultice.

BITES AND STINGS: If you've got a bite or sting that is bothering you, either apply a poultice or eat some food that contains garlic.

A WORD OF CAUTION: In rare cases, garlic can cause heartburn. This is, however, very rare. Conversely, there are studies that indicate that it cuts down on the risk of stomach cancers. Otherwise, it's perfectly safe to use.

INTERESTING FACTS: Historically, garlic has been around for thousands of years. The Roman naturalist Pliny said it was of 'great benefit against changes of water and residence', and recommended it for many ailments, including asthma. The Chinese used it for fever and dysentery. Louis Pasteur, of milk fame, noted its antibacterial qualities in 1858.

Ginger

This herb's a beauty, if you know what I mean, in herbal terms. There are only a few others to touch it when it comes to the amount of things it can do. So the first thing I'm going to say, is please refer to the glossary (page 291). I can't possibly squeeze them all in here, though I would like to. It's just that I might need the whole book! It does so much you see. That's in addition to it being a pleasant food flavouring. So I'm not going to waste any more time. Here goes!

PREVENTING HEART DISEASE: Get going with the ginger powder on your food. It's a very good, not to mention delicious, way of preventing blood clots and keeping the circulation up to scratch. What's more, ginger is also good for preventing migraines and stroke, all because of its excellent qualities.

ANGINA: Obviously, if it's so good at keeping the blood from clotting, and the heart healthy, then it has to be useful for this. That's because it strengthens the heart muscle tissue and protects the blood vessels against cholesterol damage. Quite a lot really. What's more, it needn't cost you the earth. Powdered ginger is so easy to come by and all you have to do is add a little to your meals each day to start gaining the benefit.

CHRONIC FATIGUE SYNDROME: Ginger is an antiviral herb, meaning it can help against viruses. I don't think it would work on its own with this condition but you could try adding it to your diet or taking capsules.

COUGH: Try putting some powdered ginger into your cough medicine the next time that you have a cold. It should help to suppress it.

FEVER: The same goes if you have a fever. Put a little in your tea or food. Equally, you could look for ginger tablets and keep them handy for when the need arises.

LARYNGITIS: Again, ginger tea is good for this condition, as it is for any of respiratory tract illnesses generally.

NAUSEA/MOTION SICKNESS: Everyone knows that most motion sickness tablets contain ginger. It's very good for nausea. You can even try eating the candied ginger sweet. Unlike licorice candy, which is sometimes just a flavouring, this does contain ginger.

TENDINITIS: Ginger could help this condition. It tends to reduce inflammation generally, so taking it as a tea, tablet or in your food might just ease things.

VIRAL INFECTIONS: Ginger is sometimes good against certain viral infections and, as everyone reacts differently to illnesses, it might be it could help you if you added it to your cooking.

A WORD OF CAUTION: In some instances, ginger has been known to cause miscarriage. This is only in extremely high doses, however. I'm not talking about a sprinkling on your food, or a piece of the candied variety. I'm talking about people spooning the jar down every day in life – most unlikely I would think. Obviously, as with any herb, it doesn't do to overdose, and you should take it according to the instructions that are printed on the tea packet, or capsule bottle. The latter has already been made up into safe dosages.

INTERESTING FACT: A beautiful plant in appearance, but very difficult to grow indoors here, ginger has been used as a spice and medicine for thousands of years. The Greeks, Romans, Indians all knew about ginger, although there are some questions about its exact origins.

Gingko biloba

I've heard it said that gingko biloba is the most long lived tree in the world. The most common place to find the gingko tree is America although, as you will see throughout the book, there are a great many variations of gingko biloba.

This is one of my firm favourites and one I personally take by way of a supplement every day. It has a huge range of properties that are advantageous to a huge range of ailments.

ALZHEIMER'S DISEASE: Primarily increasing the blood flow to the brain, thus preventing memory loss, patients in the early stages of Alzheimer's have found remarkable results after using gingko biloba extract. Ageing on the whole has been proven to slow down in patients using gingko biloba extracts. The theory behind this lies in studies carried out that show circulation is improved, thus allowing a more efficient flow of blood to the vital arteries.

AS AN ANTI-DEPRESSANT: I myself have successfully concluded that gingko biloba extract has been successful in some of my clients, where more conventional anti-depressants have failed, or where the client simply refuses to take medically recommended anti-depressants. I recently read an article where a stroke victim's improvement was put down to the usage of gingko biloba supplements.

VERTIGO AND BALANCE: Again, gingko biloba extracts have been found to be beneficial to patients suffering from inner ear problems, including tinnitus (ringing in the ear).

A WORD OF CAUTION: The manufacturer's guide should be followed but, on the whole, no more than 160 mg should be taken in 24 hours. While it is believed that there are no serious side effects – and I personally have never come across any, not even in pregnant woman – care should, as always, be taken with any self-prescribed drug. In fact, gingko biloba has very few, if any, side effects that we are aware of.

INTERESTING FACTS: Gingko biloba has been used for approximately 5,000 years.

I personally use gingko biloba primarily to prevent any further memory loss. (I'm renowned for my bad memory . . . when it suits me!) As a sufferer of asthma, I again feel benefit from gingko biloba.

In my line of work as a healer, I have had positive feedback from clients who have used gingko biloba for many conditions, such as depression, headaches, in particular migraines, and one client who swears gingko biloba helped her pass an exam which otherwise she felt she would have failed. Her reason for this statement was simply that her concentration had been appalling but after using gingko biloba she found her mental awareness sharpened.

Ginseng – American

American ginseng grows wild in the northern and central areas of the United States and, like its famous cousin Asian ginseng, is generally good for stress and athletic performance. Where American ginseng comes into its own, however, is in dealing with stomach problems and it is for this reason that it is cultivated in China. Extracts of it are not generally available, so it might be that you would need to consult a homeopathic doctor or dietician, or enquire at your health shop about how you could come by this, if you feel it would be beneficial to you.

A WORD OF CAUTION: If you have managed to track it down in either capsule, tablet or tincture form, I would refer to the warnings given for its cousins, Asian and Siberian, as many of the illnesses it is good for are the same.

INTERESTING FACTS: American ginseng was used by Native American tribes for digestive disorders. It was imported to China in the 1700s. Talk about taking ice to the Eskimos!

Ginseng – Asian

(Also known as Korean or Chinese ginseng)

Ginseng is one of those wonderful plants that has been around for hundreds of years and which is now being extensively studied to prove its worth, as it were. As if we takers didn't already know! Asian ginseng, which also includes the above, is cultivated in China, Korea and Japan and is useful for a variety of ailments, so many it would pay you to look up the glossary. The ones I'm concentrating on here are:

ALZHEIMER'S DISEASE: Traditionally, Asian ginseng was used to enlighten the mind and increase wisdom. It is recognised to be useful for improving the memory and, because it increases the circulation, it may help with this condition. In addition to this it is said to stop agitation, something that may be beneficial in the treatment of some sufferers.

ATHLETIC PERFORMANCE: Ginseng has also been used for thousands of years as an energy-giving tonic. Indeed, some Olympic athletes have been known to use it to keep their energy levels high and improve their alertness in a competitive situation. It does, however, take a month for people using this herb to see an improvement, so if you're an athlete and are concerned about having sufficient energy levels to cope with your particular sport, then you would have to start taking it beforehand. There's no point getting to the games and thinking, 'I'll start taking it now.'

FATIGUE: Because it is such an energy booster, ginseng can combat tiredness, although again it would take up to a month for this to take effect. It's still well worth a try if you suffer permanently from exhaustion.

IMMUNE SYSTEM: People with problems with their immune system or who seem always to catch everything that's going, should find that the compounds in ginseng will help things generally for them.

CIRCULATION: Generally ginseng increases the blood flow through the body and has been found to be useful for people with circulatory problems.

DEPRESSION: Ginseng is very good for stress, agitation and also lightening the mood. I personally recommend it for depression and have one client who has found it beneficial in his case, reporting that within two weeks of taking extracts, his mood seemed to lift.

RECUPERATION: In addition to helping with certain illnesses, ginseng is very good for getting those who are recuperating back on their feet. If you are finding the going slow for whatever reason, then you should pay a visit to the health counter in your supermarket or health shop and see what's on offer for you there.

A WORD OF CAUTION: People with uncontrolled high blood pressure should not use ginseng and neither should pregnant, breast-feeding women or people on vitamin C supplements. Because it stimulates the system, washing tablets down with coffee or tea is a bad idea, one that can lead to gastric upset. In some instances too, it can lead to insomnia. Apart from this, however, ginseng is safe when taken in the recommended dose and with the week 'off' that most manufacturers stick to. It comes as a tablet and tincture and is available from supermarkets and health shops.

INTERESTING FACTS: The use of ginseng dates to the first century AD. In Chinese medicine it was used to treat elderly people and improve their mental and physical vitality.

Ginseng - Siberian

Siberian Ginseng is a relative of Asian, a sort of shyer, not so popular, second cousin many times removed, with, in some respects, many of the same features. It was originally used to combat colds, flu and respiratory tract infections. Like its big cousin it is also used by athletes to increase their performance. Many divers and sailors used it traditionally to prevent stress-related illnesses.

As with Asian ginseng, Siberian ginseng also helps with Alzheimer's disease, fatigue, the immune system and stress.

COLDS/FLU: Siberian ginseng could well be the one to take to avoid getting flu if it's on the prowl. Research shows that one of the compounds boosts the immune system by increasing the number of immune cells in the body, thus warding off flu symptoms.

HEALTHY GLAND FUNCTION: Another benefit of Siberian ginseng is that it keeps the glands functioning properly, especially when the body is being challenged by stress. It also helps cleanse the liver of nasty toxins.

A WORD OF CAUTION: As with Asian ginseng, you should avoid this if you are pregnant, breast-feeding, or have uncontrolled high blood pressure. Also, avoid taking it at bedtime, as it can lead to insomnia. In some people it can cause diarrhoea. Siberian ginseng is available from your health shop and comes as a tincture, powdered capsules and dried root.

INTERESTING FACTS: Siberian ginseng is also known as devil's shrub. It was given to many Russian and Ukrainian people after Chernobyl to counteract the effects of radiation.

Green tea

When it was first suggested a few years ago that tea was good for preventing cancer, there was a sort of general stampede to the tea alley in the supermarket to pick up the latest from Typhoo and we were all to be heard anxiously reeling off exactly how many times a day we did it – drink tea that is.

Of course, one thing many of us didn't pick up on was that it wasn't just any old tea. Your plain PG or Earl Grey just wasn't enough, although that's not to say they don't have their own qualities and aren't useful in other ways.

Green tea, however, was the one that was attracting all the attention. It's made from the same plant, of course, but rolled and dried differently, in order to preserve the substances. The leaves that go into your average cuppa have been fermented, thus removing many of the therapeutic ingredients. Products bearing the name gunpowder tea are 'green', however. I have many clients who don't think they are too fiery and have certainly survived taking them!

GINGIVITIS: Gingivitis, along with other gum diseases such as pyorrhoea and mouth ulcers, should begin to subside if you take green tea, combined with three or four days of high doses of vitamin C.

GENERAL GOOD HEALTH: The presence of fluoride, tannins and catechins, means that green tea sipped regularly may help prevent heart disease, ageing, certain types of cancer and tooth decay. It is also known to boost the immune system and reduce or even prevent infection. Green tea is easily available from all health food shops and is therefore an easy and pleasant way to enjoy a cup of tea on a daily basis and thus help to maintain all-round good health, or at least we stand a better chance of having all-round good health.

STOMACH UPSET: A cup of green tea can help soothe an upset stomach.

GENERAL RELAXATION: Green tea is even getting in on the beauty stakes and is now available, along with other herbs, as a fragrant bath soak and also an eye cream.

A WORD OF CAUTION: If you have a particularly sensitive stomach, the tannin in green tea can cause irritation. Take the tea with milk to reduce any ill affects. Pregnant women should avoid green tea and take green tea supplements instead. The caffeine content is high – about 40 mg to a cup – and can cause slow foetal growth. The same goes if you have a weak heart, kidney disease, anxiety, panic attacks, or are breast-feeding. Supplements, however, contain only 5 mg of caffeine in a 125 mg pill, thus making it much safer to take. Also, never drink green tea when it is very hot, as this does harm to the throat. It can also cause insomnia if taken too near to bedtime

INTERESTING FACTS: Legend has it that a Chinese emperor was drinking hot water when some leaves from a nearby tea shrub dropped in the cup. We believe it! There would be no such thing as elevenses otherwise! The Chinese believe that green tea is beneficial in a great many situations, from treating pain to prolonging life, from depression to digestion.

Hawthorn

The qualities of the hawthorn tree were originally recognised by the ancient Greeks and Native Americans centuries ago and although Britain was slower to follow on, our Victorian ancestors would certainly have included some in their medical cabinets.

Hawthorn is now a frequently prescribed heart remedy in Europe. One that works by opening up the blood vessels that feed the heart, thus increasing its power. Hawthorn also decreases blood cholesterol levels and blood pressure, relieving strain on the heart.

ANGINA: Using the recommended dose of 100–150 mg three times a day, hawthorn is a powerful heart medicine. However, due to the enormity of this condition I would recommend that you first discuss with your doctor whether or not to use hawthorn (or any other supplement), especially if you are already on prescription medicines. Research shows that hawthorn may be a good preventative, but nothing has been proven, as yet, to show whether it will stop an acute attack of angina.

AS A HEART TONIC: Where hawthorn comes into its own is as a heart tonic. By increasing the blood flow, it also increases the heart's ability to cope with a loss of oxygen, which is what happens when the coronary arteries become clogged. By keeping the heart beating properly it helps prevent heart fatigue. Thus it can be seen as a preventative medicine for those who feel they may be at risk from heart disease.

AVAILABILITY: Hawthorn can be taken in many forms – as a tincture, tablet, powder, tea or capsule – all of which should be available at your local health store.

A WORD OF CAUTION: None have been recorded. However, heart defects are serious and should never be self-treated.

INTERESTING FACT: Hawthorn was often planted in hedges to keep human intruders at bay. Its prickly branches were an ideal deterrent for trespassers. The old saying, 'Ne'er cast a clout till May is out,' does not refer to the month but the appearance of the hawthorn ('May blossom') flowers.

Homeopathy

WHAT IS IT? Homeopathy is a bit like immunisation. It works by giving patients a small dose of a substance that creates the same symptoms as the illness. The substance is largely mineral or herbal, of course, rather than chemical and it is then diluted to suit.

HOW DOES IT WORK? A properly prepared remedy will be geared to the individual, not just the disease. This is important because everyone's response to an illness is different. Even when you think about the common cold, one person might just sneeze a little and have a runny nose, while someone else might be absolutely floored and have to take to their bed. A qualified homeopath will take a case study of your illness, diet and your feelings about your illness, before suggesting what is best for you, so the medicine they come up with is likely to help. Having said that, you can buy certain remedies over the counter for some of the 'minor' ailments, such as hayfever or a cold – things that are an irritant to you.

WHAT DOES IT HELP IN PARTICULAR? All kinds of 'minor' type ailments from allergies to migraines.

HOW LONG SHOULD A COURSE OF TREATMENT LAST? Obviously this depends on a number of things, e.g. your illness, whether you buy a remedy over the counter or go to a trained homeopath, and on the remedy itself. Some are meant to be taken every few hours for a certain period of time. Others can be daily for a few weeks. This is very much a 'horses for courses' therapy. You might find that what you are taking isn't working so it might be necessary to try something else, thus involving a different dosage altogether.

HOW DO I GO ABOUT GETTING THIS TREATMENT? Remedies are available at health shops or you can see a qualified homeopath. Ask at your health shop.

A WORD OF CAUTION: Obviously you must make sure that the condition you are seeking advice about is that condition and not something else, otherwise the medicine won't help and your health may be suffering because you haven't had your illness properly diagnosed in the first place. If you are pregnant check with your doctor first. Most remedies contain small amounts of alcohol, so this is something to think about if you don't drink. Make sure your practitioner is properly qualified and that you follow the instructions on whatever remedy they suggest or you purchase, if it is of the over-the-counter, self-help variety.

INTERESTING FACT: Homeopathy has been around a few hundred years. It is the work of a German chemist and doctor Samme Hahnemann who got rather fed up with the conventional medicine of the time. Since that involved purging and blood letting, who can blame him for trying a few alternatives? And these must have worked. He lived to be 90!

Honeysuckle

The flowers of this plant aren't just nice to look at, smell or make up songs about. They contain many antiseptic compounds and traditionally have been used for problems associated with the respiratory tract. If you're a regular sufferer of any of the following then ask at your health shop for products containing honeysuckle and make them part of your medicine cabinet, or plant your own honeysuckle. I would think it'd be bound to help.

BRONCHITIS: Either ask at your health shop or make your own honeysuckle tea by pouring a cup of boiling water on a handful of petals and straining them before drinking. The antiseptic compounds should soon soothe your throat and cool the 'fire' in your chest. Take two cups a day.

COLDS AND FLU: Again, taking honeysuckle tea or other preparations containing honeysuckle extracts will help you over the worst of this.

SORE THROAT: This is where honeysuckle comes into its own, soon acting against the bacteria that can cause a sore throat. Ask at your health shop for an extract and keep it handy for use if you feel a sore throat coming on. The sooner the compounds have the chance to get to work, the sooner you'll feel better. Remember that some sore throats can affect the whole system, leaving you feeling very run down. Not worth risking, I'd say.

TONSILLITIS: Okay, tonsillitis is in a class of its own when it comes to sore throat, and not a class I particularly like being in myself. But because honeysuckle is so effective against sore throat, I'd be more than willing to try it for this condition, too.

PNEUMONIA: Of course, if you have this condition, you don't mess about. You might find that honeysuckle tea aids your recovery, however.

A WORD OF CAUTION: Do make sure that the flower you are pouring boiling water on *is* honeysuckle, if you decide to go down this route, and not some other plant you think might be honeysuckle! I know that sounds silly but sometimes our knowledge of plants isn't all it could be and many are toxic. Honeysuckle isn't, however, and I personally have never come across anyone who has experienced ill effects using it. I wouldn't like you to be the first because you're using something that's not it though! So please be careful.

INTERESTING FACTS: Honeysuckle is named after a sixteenth-century botanist. It is used widely in Chinese medicine for all of the above.

Horse chestnut

Good old horse chestnut, useful for so many things, as well as being a lovely tree. Horse chestnut was used traditionally to treat many things, including arthritis and pain and may still be good for these. Europeans use it widely for the treatment of sports injuries and sprain. The seeds are rich in aescin, a substance that increases circulation generally. When applied locally it has also been known to reduce oedema.

HAEMORRHOIDS: Taking horse chestnut orally can actually increase constipation, thus making this condition worse, but a gel containing either horse chestnut or aescin, the substance that it contains, can certainly help reduce pain and swelling. Ask at your health shop for one.

PAIN AND SPRAIN: The same goes for this. You can even buy a tincture and make a poultice to apply to the injured area. Horse chestnut is very good for treating sprain, so a bandage soaked in the tincture and water might help reduce swelling. If you're doing this, add a little witch hazel. The two work wonders when combined.

VARICOSE VEINS: Again, applying aescin gel or tincture on a poultice (see above) can help this aggravating condition. Remember to follow instructions carefully and to use the gel as directed. Although it is safe to take two or three drops of tincture, not enough aescin can be absorbed this way, so stick to a gel, then it works directly on the skin.

WRINKLES: You might find the gel is also useful for creaming away or at least reducing wrinkles. Just watch your eyes. Any cream in the eye can be dangerous and we don't want to be looking up the remedy for that now, do we?

A WORD OF CAUTION: Horse chestnut should be avoided by people with kidney or liver disease, although it is perfectly safe when given to those with healthy organs. Nor does it cause damage to these organs. It is generally regarded as safe to take if you are pregnant. Sometimes it can cause itching, and nausea if taken orally.

INTERESTING FACTS: Traditionally, horse chestnut leaves were used to treat fevers. The horse in the name has nothing to do with animals. Horses won't eat the fruit of this tree. It means inferior and refers to the wood, which isn't much use for making things, as the tree grows so quickly, and also the 'conker', or fruit, which is thought to be inferior to the sweet chestnut. Another name for the horse chestnut is the candle tree.

Iodine

Iodine is one of those little healers our mothers used to keep to hand in the first aid kit, which has been ignored a bit of late. It is, however, an excellent antiseptic for bacterial skin conditions, killing the germs on impact. Keep a bottle handy in the cupboard. You might like to use it for:

CUTS: Just don't put it on the open wound! If you remember, what our mothers used to do was paint round the problem, avoiding the cut itself! It's antiseptic action goes to work immediately to stop any infection spreading.

INFLAMMATION: If a wound has sealed but the area around it is red and inflamed, carefully apply a little iodine on a tissue. You should soon see a difference.

CORNS: Paint corns nightly with Iodine to help them disperse.

BOILS: If a boil is coming up, swab it three times a day to stop it developing. Paint round it to bring it to a head.

A WORD OF CAUTION: Do not overuse! Iodine has serious side effects if you absorb too much into your blood. Never apply it to open wounds, deep cuts, ulcerated skin, or near the eyes. If you are pregnant or nursing don't use iodine and, although it is good for treating irritations, don't use on babies under one month old. Otherwise, used as instructed, iodine is not expected to produce any side effects. On occasion it can cause irritation where a user is allergic. If that happens, discontinue use.

INTERESTING FACT: Strong iodine is sometimes prescribed orally for an over-active thyroid gland.

Ipriflavone

Ipriflavone is a bit of a mouthful to say and a bit of a headache to explain in terms of what it is. But what it does is helpful. If you want to have healthy bones, read on. That's what it's mainly about.

Ipriflavone is a derivative that that comes from compounds found in soy beans and other plants, a sort of a bit of a bit, if you know what I mean, and has recently become available in supplement form.

OSTEOPOROSIS: Small, thin women are most at risk of developing osteoporosis, or weakening of the bones. But women in general are more at risk of developing this condition, particularly after the menopause.

Ipriflavone supplements help maintain the density of the bone and guard against fractures. Its bone strengthening effect can be enhanced by taking calcium and vitamin D along with it. A two-year study involving Italian women showed that those who took supplements without calcium, experienced significant bone loss, while those taking both maintained bone density.

A WORD OF CAUTION: If you have asthma, emphysema or other lung disorder, consult your doctor before taking ipriflavone, as it can react negatively with certain medicines. Don't take it when you are pregnant or breast-feeding, if you have a liver or kidney disorder, or are suffering breast cancer.

INTERESTING FACT: Although relatively new to the UK, Japanese and European women have known of its benefits for some time.

Ivy

Okay, so own up! You thought ivy was just a tiresome weed that strangles everything in sight in your garden, or something someone once wrote a Christmas carol about. Well, it's not. Ivy is an old folk remedy, often overlooked these days. Traditionally, it was used for throat problems and respiratory problems. So, if you're a sufferer, you should pay a visit to your local health shop and see what's there for you containing ivy. It has expectorant qualities, meaning it loosens up these secretions, which makes you cough.

BRONCHITIS: If you suffer from bronchitis, then ask at your health shop. Any preparation containing ivy should help to ease the respiratory tract.

COUGH: A pinch of dried ivy can relieve a cough, even whooping cough. If you can't find a preparation containing ivy at your local health store, then you should be able to buy it dried. Add it to your normal cough medicine.

LARYNGITIS: It is possible that ivy could help ease this condition, because of the qualities it contains.

SKIN PROBLEMS: Since ivy contains saponin, an anti-fungal compound, you can certainly try using it to treat dermatitis. You can even chop up some of you own ivy leaves if you've got any. Blend them with a little water and apply the resulting paste to the affected area.

CANDIDA: A cup of ivy tea helps fight yeast infections. Just put a pinch of dried herb, obtainable from your health shop, in a cup of boiling water for ten minutes, strain, then drink.

A WORD OF CAUTION: None that I can think of, providing you are using ivy according to instructions. Personally speaking, having recently taken up gardening, I now find I am beginning to detest the stuff. It just seems to appear everywhere – even when I can see no sign of any ivy bush or root!

INTERESTING FACTS: There are over 50 species of ivy. Ivy was occasionally planted in graveyards to give the imitation of grass. The common Irish ivy often grows beneath yew trees, where grass will not live.

Juniper

Evergreen juniper trees can be found all over the world and although we talk of juniper berries and I refer to making tea with them, they are actually the dark blue scales from the pine cones of the tree.

URINARY TRACT INFECTIONS: The oils in juniper act as a diuretic, flushing out bacteria from the bladder, so may help relieve annoying urinary infections. You can try taking it in tablet form as per instruction, or make a tea. Very often juniper is combined with other diuretic herbs. Ask at your health store for details.

COLDS AND FLU: The compounds in juniper act against colds and even flu. So if you feel one coming on, you can think about taking some tablets or tea with juniper in them. They may not cure the virus but they should ease away some of the symptoms. Since some of these compounds also work against herpes sores, taking juniper could prevent cold sores from developing – often a hard-to-cure side effect of viral infections of this type.

AVAILABILITY: Juniper tablets and tinctures are available from your health shop. Always read the dosage carefully. To make a tea, you can steep a teaspoonful of berries to a cup of boiling water, in a tightly covered container.

A WORD OF CAUTION: Juniper should be avoided if you are pregnant

– just think of all those old wives' tales about gin and the bath tub and you will know why. Check the instructions to see that what you are taking does not interact with other medicines. Anyone with serious kidney disease should not take juniper at all. It has been known to cause damage with some people. Because of this please don't take juniper for long periods of time. Its benefits are for short-term illness only, not to help health in general, as I have suggested with other remedies. The fact it causes kidney damage in some people is enough to make me cautious. I might be one of these people! However, there is no reason not to use it for the things it is best at.

INTERESTING FACT: As well as being used to flavour gin – very medicinal I am sure! – juniper was traditionally used as a perfume and for making soap. I have my own supply at hand for my 'weighing in' days at my slimming club! As a diuretic, it can make all the difference on those dreaded scales!

Lavender

Many years ago, when I was having trouble sleeping, a friend recommended using a lavender pillow. Since then I've had great respect for this lovely herb and all its many uses. One of the best things about it is that you can grow your own so easily. As well as adding a pleasant smell to your garden, you'll find lavender can benefit your health in a variety of ways and, although it can sometimes cause nausea if taken internally, it is very safe to use on the skin. So let's take a look at some of the things you'll be digging up your garden for if you decide to plant a clump. Well worth it, I'm sure.

BURNS: Placing lavender oil on a burn can soothe and heal the damaged skin. Please note the word 'placing'. While it is safe to take a few drops in tincture form, you should never take lavender oil as it can be toxic.

FAINTING: Keep a small sachet of dried lavender and rosemary in your pocket, then if someone faints you can go gallantly to the rescue. Victorian ladies used to faint all the time, usually because their corsets were too tight. That's why so many of them carried lavender sachets. If you grow the plant, you can make your own.

INSOMNIA: Sprinkling lavender oil on your pillow, or buying a lavender pillow, can help give you a good night's rest. I should know. If you're buying the oil, ask at your health store for one that's soothing – some can actually stimulate the senses.

PAIN: Traditionally, lavender oil was used to treat headaches and rheumatism. Keeping a small jar of lavender oil in your medicine cabinet could be useful. A few drops can be safely mixed with vegetable oil, then massaged onto the sore area, or alternatively soaked onto a small cloth and held against it.

VAGINITIS: Adding a few drops of oil to a bath may help soothe this condition. But please don't try rubbing it on this area, unless you want real problems.

PREGNANCY: Sometimes when you're pregnant you can feel tired and depressed, especially as the months go on. Bathing regularly in lavender oil or drinking lavender tea can help beat the former. To make the tea you steep a teaspoon of leaves in a cup of boiling water for 15 minutes. Two cups can be drunk a day. Taking a bath in lavender oil can help after you've had the baby too. Lavender can soothe and reduce the discomfort we all know about but don't like to mention!

STRESS: Traditionally, herbalists used lavender to treat fatigue, so it may well be helpful here. You can try burning some lavender oil, adding some to a bath, or even tossing a handful of stalks from your own plant into the water at the end of the day. Remember, stress is often the result of how we live, so don't expect one lavender scented bath to work wonders. Looking at your whole life as a whole, and trying to find ways of changing it, is just as important. However, you should find that using lavender will have a generally calming effect. I personally love lavender shower gel and use it every day!

AVAILABILITY: Lavender can be grown, bought as an oil, or look for perfume and bath products containing it.

A WORD OF CAUTION: Never take the oil.

INTERESTING FACT: A French perfume chemist gets the credit for inventing aromatherapy. When he burnt his hand he plunged it into the nearest container, which happened to contain lavender oil. Apparently the hand healed with no scarring. The rest, as they say, is history.

Lemon grass

We tend to think of this as a food flavouring and very nice it is too. But it's another of those herbs that have uses over and above that. In South America, Africa and Asia, lemon grass has been a popular folk remedy for centuries and is used for a variety of different ailments. So perhaps it's time we cottoned on.

ATHLETE'S FOOT: The essential oil has been found to have anti-fungal properties so, obviously, it's a first stop for this one. You can try mixing a teaspoon of the oil with one of vegetable oil and dabbing it on the affected area as often as necessary until it has cleared. Your other option is to put the leaves in a basin of boiling water, allow to steep for ten minutes, then put you foot in. Just make sure the water has cooled down first or you'll have scalded feet to add to your troubles! In fact, I think you'll find that lemon grass is helpful for fungal infections of the skin generally.

FEVER/COUGH/FLU: In Latin American countries lemon grass is used to treat these three ailments. Just steep one teaspoon of dried herb in a cup of hot water for ten minutes. Strain, then drink. Repeat three times a day until you feel better.

UPSET STOMACH: Lemon grass tea is also widely used in Africa, South America and Asia to soothe an upset stomach and dispense wind. It's particularly good if your upset is down to nerves, tension or anxiety, which many are. But its antiseptic qualities also make it useful for calming any queasiness caused by bacteria.

A WORD OF CAUTION: So far as I can gather there are no noted cautions regarding the use of this herb. The only real problem is the way it tends to be viewed in the UK, and that is as a food flavouring. This means you would have to 'make your own', so to speak, in terms of a tea, but if you have the dried herb to hand that shouldn't be a problem.

INTERESTING FACT: Lemon grass is related to citronella and has the same insect-repelling qualities.

Licorice

I really wouldn't like to list all the things licorice is good for – I could be here all day! But since this is a book about health care, I suppose I'm going to have to! To find out more you must refer to the glossary (page 292) because licorice is one of those amazing things that contains so many substances. The list is endless and unfortunately this book isn't! However, here are just a few to give you a taste of it, so to speak! And you thought it was just a sweet!

SHINGLES, ECZEMA, PSORIASIS: Licorice cream is ideal for treating any of these conditions. That's because it contains substances that reduce inflammation, itching and burning. For some reason, too, it boosts the effectiveness of other creams. Quite amazing really! Either ask at your health shop or buy a licorice tea and apply it to the rash.

FATIGUE: Now here's another amazing fact. There's nothing new about chronic fatigue. If you look at my section on anaemia (page 15) you'll see my comments on a type of fatigue that existed a hundred years ago, which some researchers think is exactly what is on the go today. And the medicine that was recommended for it was – yes, you've guessed it – licorice extract. That's because it can ease stress and increase energy levels throughout the body. So what are you waiting for? If this is a problem for you, get down to your health shop and buy some.

ASTHMA, EMPHYSEMA, SORE THROAT, CONGESTION: All these conditions can be soothed by taking licorice, either as an extract, tea, lozenge or tincture. Licorice can reduce coughing spasms, soothe airways and loosen mucus. Not bad at all I say.

PMS, MENSTRUATION, MENOPAUSAL PROBLEMS: Licorice has been shown to help reduce symptoms of irritability and bloating as well as minimising menopausal symptoms associated with a decline in oestrogen.

HEART DISEASE: Studies show that 100 mg a day can help prevent the arteries from clogging, thus keeping the heart functioning properly.

IMMUNE SYSTEM: Again, studies show that one of the substances in licorice can boost the immune system, helping to prevent breast and colon cancer.

DANDRUFF: The same substance, believe it or not, can help control dandruff of all things! Keep a handful of the dried herb in vinegar and apply it when needed.

A WORD OF CAUTION: Licorice is a very powerful and beneficial herb. The amount of things it can help shows that it contains substances that need to be handled carefully. Although you might think of it as just a sweet, it's not. In fact there are a lot of cautions, particularly to do with other medications and dosage. So let's look at them.

Don't take licorice if you take blood pressure drugs, steroids or are on diuretics. It interferes with these drugs and the system. Licorice can actually raise blood pressure. So if you're taking it for more than four weeks, you should have your blood pressure checked. In high doses, over long periods of time, licorice can also cause headache, swelling, stiffness, shortage of breath, lethargy and heart irregularity. In fact it can cause all the things it seeks to cure, so use it wisely according to the instructions and don't overdose on it. You should also avoid licorice if you have an eating disorder, are pregnant or breast-feeding, have diabetes or already have diseases of the liver, heart or kidneys. Avoid combining licorice candy and soft drinks with licorice supplements as this may confuse the dosage and raise your blood pressure. Goodness!

However, if you take it according to the instructions and don't suffer any of these conditions, you should find it's a good and beneficial herbal medicine to use.

INTERESTING FACTS: Licorice has been used for hundreds of years. It is widely cultivated in Greece and Turkey. Research is currently ongoing into its many diverse healing properties.

Linseed oil

This sounds like something you stick on the garden furniture to preserve it. Well, you can. But the stuff I'm talking about here, is the vegetable oil that gives us one of the essential fatty acids we all need for survival. It's not suitable for cooking though, so don't get any ideas about suddenly converting it to that. However, it can be used in salads and small amounts are found in certain foodstuffs – walnut oils, blackcurrants and soya are a few. Some research shows that it lowers the blood pressure, so if you're a sufferer from high blood pressure, it could be helpful.

CONSTIPATION: If you're a sufferer you can try putting a tablespoonful of the oil on a salad, in order to get things going. Obviously, if your constipation continues and nothing at all seems to be working, see your doctor.

VAGINITIS: If you suffer regularly from this condition then it might be a good idea to add linseed oil to your diet generally to improve things. You can try putting it on salad, or vegetables.

A WORD OF CAUTION: Although some studies suggest that large amounts of linseed oil may increase cancer risks, the link is far from conclusive. As with all things, use in moderation. You'll note I'm not saying 'ladle it in the salad' here. Be sensible.

INTERESTING FACT: Actual deficiencies of the fatty oil that linseed oil contains are rare.

Magnesium

Magnesium is very necessary for making new cells, activating the B vitamins, blood clotting, regulating the heart, relaxing muscles, keeping the bones healthy, giving us protein and forming the fatty acids. Will I go on? Well, yes, because not enough attention has been paid to the vital role magnesium plays in keeping us healthy. There are studies that suggest people with chronic fatigue syndrome and children with attention deficit disorder have low levels of magnesium in their bodies. Equally, there are some that don't. Which just goes to show, you can't account for all the people all of the time! Seriously, I take the view that because we are all so different, different things work for different people. And when you're ill with certain conditions, you're desperate too. Therefore anything is worth a try and discussing with your doctor. Foodwise, magnesium is found in nuts, coriander, lettuce, dark green vegetables, fish and meat – oh – and beans by the way. I mention that last because of the side effect they sometimes have! But people who are seriously deficient often need intravenous treatment rather than eating up their dark greens, or taking oral supplements. The signs are fatigue, muscle weakness, listlessness and loss of appetite. You are also more likely to be deficient if you have had a severe burn, are diabetic, take too many laxatives all the time, or suffer from alcoholism. If you are suffering chronic fatigue, regular migraines, or have a child with ADHD (attention-deficit hyperactivity disorder), it is certainly worth discussing the possibility of a serious deficiency with your doctor. What I am doing below is taking a look at other conditions that can benefit from increasing your magnesium levels. Because we eat so much processed food in the UK it's likely that quite a lot of us aren't getting enough magnesium, and that's a pity.

ANGINA: Having good magnesium levels can help promote a healthy heart. If you suffer from angina, or are worried about developing a heart condition, then think about what I've said above. Magnesium keeps blood pressure down by relaxing the muscles. If your magnesium levels are low, then your heart will suffer.

HEADACHE: Some nutritionists think we don't get enough magnesium in our diet and that a deficiency can lead to headaches. If you suffer headaches often, or experience frequent migraines, then it may be you need to up your levels. Try increasing the amount of magnesium foods in your diet, or taking supplements, which are available from your health shop or supermarket. Serious deficiencies should be taken up with your doctor

FATIGUE: Fatigue is a sign of low magnesium levels. If you're tired more frequently than usual, then taking a supplement may help this, as will eating more dark green vegetables. Spinach is very good here – Popeye the sailor wasn't joking – but so are lettuce and coriander.

ASTHMA/BRONCHITIS: Both these conditions can be linked to a drop in magnesium levels, in that the risk of an attack increases as the levels fall. So keep on eating the foods I've mentioned if you want to help prevent these occurring.

TENDINITIS: Since magnesium is such a good mineral for bones and muscles, regularly eating foods that contain it can help keep them healthy. Okay, if you use a particular joint all the time, the chances are it will become inflamed, but if you do suffer this condition then you can always try taking a supplement in addition to your diet in order to fight it.

A WORD OF CAUTION: Although the amounts found in supplements are too low to cause problems, taking too much magnesium can lead to diarrhoea. This can vary from person to person. If you have kidney disease you shouldn't take supplements without seeing your doctor first. Always take any supplement according to the instructions and stop if it seems to be disagreeing with you. Also, remember to be patient if you start taking supplements or adding magnesium foods to your diet. It takes weeks for levels to build up.

INTERESTING FACT: Almost two thirds of people in intensive care units have a magnesium deficiency. Now that's food for thought!

Marsh mallow

'Once widely used in medicine, mallows are no longer considered of value.' No, I didn't write that. I'm just quoting from a source of 50 years ago and thinking how short sighted! Particularly if you look along the shelves of your local health shop or supermarket. Marsh mallow has certainly made a comeback, which just goes to show, you can't keep a good thing down, or indeed ignore the work it has done for hundreds of years. Among other things, these include:

COLDS AND FLU: Marsh mallow has been used for thousands of years to treat colds and flu. The roots contain a substance that soothes inflammation, particularly of the mucous membranes. I'm not suggesting digging up a mallow plant to help your cold, however! Look for preparations containing it at your health shop and keep them handy for when you have a cold.

BRONCHITIS: Similarly, I think you'll find that marsh mallow will also help sufferers from this condition. (See 'Colds and flu' above.)

BLADDER INFECTIONS: Dried marsh mallow can help ease a bladder infection. Simply soak two tablespoonfuls in one litre of water overnight. Sip the tea through the day. Alternatively, ask at your health shop for a tincture containing it.

HEARTBURN/INDIGESTION: Camomile and marsh mallow tea is good for soothing the digestion. Either look for one that has both or add a few marsh mallow flowers to a cup of camomile. Strain and leave to cool.

VOMITING: Similarly, a tea made from marsh mallow can help stop this problem, so it's a good one to have handy in the cupboard in case anyone has a bad stomach upset.

LACTATION: Marsh mallow was traditionally used to help the milk to flow and also ease any hardening of the breasts due to mastitis. You can either make a compress from the flowers, or buy a tea. This can be both taken and used to soothe by simply putting it on a cloth. Marsh mallow also comes in tablet form, often with other herbs. Look in your health shop or supermarket.

A WORD OF CAUTION: So far as I know, marsh mallow is safe to use and I can't think of anyone having ill effects, when taken according to instructions.

INTERESTING FACT: The marsh mallow comes from the same family as the hollyhock. The mallow mentioned in the bible is thought to be the Jew's mallow.

Meadowsweet

Meadowsweet flowers are more sweat than sweet. They have been used down the centuries to cure fever and might, therefore, be useful if you have a cold or flu. The root, too, was sometimes used in tincture form. Some of the compounds react with the body to produce aspirin-like effects, making it a good herbal substitute. So far, however, the knowledge of most of meadowsweet's capabilities is based on historical use. Insufficient studies have been done in regard to its healing powers. That doesn't mean it's not worth a try. In fact you might find it useful for certain things.

FEVER: If you've got a cold or flu and your temperature has shot up, with all the misery that brings, you could try drinking a cup of tea with a teaspoon of meadowsweet flowers in it, or ask at your health shop if they have any cold remedies with meadowsweet in it. As I say so often, be prepared. There's no point waiting till a cold, then a fever, has struck. You won't be able to get out then and you'll be at the mercy of whatever your local shop has. If you're making a tea with the flowers, continue taking it till the cold symptoms have disappeared.

ULCERS: Some herbalists recommend taking meadowsweet for ulcers. Although it is similar to aspirin and some of the compounds in aspirin can cause ulcers, meadowsweet also contains other compounds that give an anti-ulcer effect. If you're not sure, consult your doctor, or ask at your health shop for a tincture and take it according to the instructions.

A WORD OF CAUTION: If you have any kind of sensitivity to aspirin then don't use meadowsweet. Do not give meadowsweet to children. If they have a fever, find something else.

INTERESTING FACT: Historically, meadowsweet was used for treating arthritis and as a diuretic.

Meditation

WHAT IS IT? Okay, so you know when you're a bit stressed. The car won't start, the phone's ringing, the Hoover/lawn mower has just popped its venerable and ancient clogs, the kids are squawking over who looked squint at who, there's a suspicious smell coming from the fridge, which you reckon is the remains of last month's vegetable curry you popped in there and (guess what) forgot about, your partner's run off with the milk-man/lollypop lady and you had an important meeting, like, ten minutes ago. And you start to breathe deeply and you chant. What you chant doesn't matter. It could be 'I can do it', it could be something not printable here. In fact it's more likely to be something not printable here. Well, surprise surprise, isn't it good to know you're indulging in the techniques of meditation? Okay, all you purists out there – sort of indulging. Meditation is not quite as I described it. It does, however, involve you sitting comfortably with your back straight, eyes closed and breathing deeply. Then you repeat a word – a mantra – to yourself, thus helping you become more in touch with yourself, calmer, less distracted so, of course, your car always starts, your kids never squawk, you remember what's in the fridge and of course your partner thinks you're such a wonderful, capable person, how could they even look at someone else? Not quite. I think you can guess I'm joking again. But meditation does have benefits for the health and works, as many other therapies do, by getting the mind in tune with the body, thus inducing mental and physical tranquillity.

HOW DOES IT WORK? With meditation you focus your thoughts and breathing to achieve a state of calm. And this holds good whether you are practising Transcendental Meditation (TM),

Mindfulness Meditation (MM), or Breathing Meditation (BM). By saying the mantra (TM) you stop distracting thoughts coming into your mind, thus allowing yourself to relax. MM helps you become more in touch with your body and mind as it happens. You pay attention to your thoughts but observe them without judgement. You also scan the body by thinking of each part, then letting go of the images associated with it. This has been found to be useful for people with chronic pain. BM involves concentrating on your breathing.

WHAT DOES IT HELP IN PARTICULAR? Some studies have shown that people who practice meditation have lower blood pressure afterwards, so it could be good for those with high blood pressure. It's also good for those with heart disease, stress, insomnia, tension headache, irritable bowel syndrome, PMT and depression. Generally, meditation has been associated with a longer life span and fewer hospitalisations. Sounds not too bad to me!

HOW LONG SHOULD A COURSE OF TREATMENT LAST? The recommended goal here is two 20-minute sessions per day. Those should ideally be before breakfast and bedtime. Practice makes perfect, apparently, and makes you more adept at achieving a state of calm. If you want to go to a class, these generally last about an hour, once a week.

HOW DO I GO ABOUT GETTING THIS TREATMENT? This is one that's easily practised at home. You can even teach yourself through videos tapes and books. Sometimes classes are offered at community centres. If you can't find a meditation class locally, and, let's be honest, sometimes they are a trifle hard to come by, you can look for a yoga class that concentrates more on the techniques of meditation than exercise. Some health centres and health shops do keep lists of practitioners, however, so check there first.

A WORD OF CAUTION: Meditation is not a cure, so if the things that drove you to take it up, such as fatigue, chronic pain, or shortness of breath, don't go away, please see your doctor. As with some other therapies, too, you might not be suited to meditation. So if you find you just can't achieve the golden tranquillity everyone else in the class seems to be raving about, give it up. It's not for you and there's absolutely no point stressing yourself out by persisting. Sometimes being in deep states of meditation can cause people to become aware of buried childhood traumas. If this happens and disturbing memories haunt you, consult a doctor. Please be aware, too, that some meditation classes have religious overtones. Look for one you're happy with.

INTERESTING FACT: Like yoga, meditation has been practised for thousands of years, mainly in India, Japan and China. It only really became a household word in the West when the Maharishi Mahesh Yogi brought it to America. I suppose, at a push, you could credit The Beatles with sort of bringing it here!

Milk thistle

Milk thistle grows wild and can be found along roadsides, fields and ditches. It is, however, the seeds of the dried flower that are used for healing purposes, so don't get any ideas about setting out to pick a few for yourself, unless you want a nasty sting and then have to refer to that section of this book! That said, milk thistle does have some uses for treating certain conditions and can be safely used, even by pregnant women.

PSORIASIS: Because milk thistle contains anti-inflammatory compounds it could be useful for treating this condition. It would do no harm to try.

LIVER PROBLEMS: This is where milk thistle really comes into its own. Compounds from the plant can help protect the liver against toxic damage, e.g. from alcohol, and can even regenerate cells. It acts by blocking the toxins and generally removing them. It also alters bile makeup, thereby reducing the risk of gallstones. To keep the liver healthy, therefore, even if you don't suffer the above, and don't over indulge, it would be a good idea to take it.

AVAILABILITY: Milk thistle is obtainable in tablet form from your health store.

A WORD OF CAUTION: Milk thistle is very safe to take although if you are on other medication check with your doctor first.

INTERESTING FACT: Milk thistle has been used for 2,000 years.

Mint (spearmint)

Talking of mint is a little confusing, because so many herbs already mentioned in this book belong to the mint family. And not just those with mint in the name, like catmint and peppermint. Basil is also a mint, as are rosemary and melissa. The mint family does sound a bit like everyone else's! And I would refer you to the appropriate sections if you want to see what these mints can do. I'm just looking at plain mint here, the kind you probably have in your garden, which is also known as spearmint. Told you it was confusing! It's very popular for culinary purposes. But traditionally it was used for medicinal ones.

HEARTBURN: Like peppermint, mint is very good for heartburn. You can buy a tea from many supermarkets and health shops and I would recommend doing this and keeping it handy, so if you're troubled, you can make yourself a cup. Or if you have mint in the garden, then pick a handful of leaves and brew yourself a cup by pouring hot water on and leaving it to stand for ten minutes, straining and drinking. A little touch of basil or sage – both mints – can also help.

MORNING SICKNESS: Mint has a very strong smell, so it's possibly worth breathing in some of the vapours if you suffer from this. Pour boiling water on a good handful of mint leaves and inhale. Certain mints – peppermint in particular – can sometimes bring on a miscarriage. Because of this I don't recommend taking the mint.

A WORD OF CAUTION: As I've said above, and many times before, please follow the advice and individual instructions for each herb. Mint is so widely used in cooking, it's not likely to do you any harm. In fact, it's very good for the digestion. But everyone is different and if you experience any reaction at all it's always best to find something else.

INTERESTING FACT: If cheese is rubbed with mint it stops it going mouldy.

Myrrh

So we all know the story of the wise men and their not so little gifts. Myrrh is, alas, the only one to feature here and it's quite unlikely it was given in plant form. I can't see the Baby Jesus being terribly pleased with that unless he was aiming for a career on *Gardener's World*. His description of lilies, mind you, might have indicated he was. Myrrh is the name given not only to the plant but also to the highly perfumed resin that comes from the plant. In addition to its aromatic qualities, it possesses a number of healing compounds. In particular it is good for:

SORE THROATS: If you can get myrrh tincture then do so and keep it in your cupboard. Two or three drops added to a little water make a useful gargle when you have a sore throat.

PREVENTING TOOTH DECAY: Again, rinsing your mouth regularly with the same mixture can help prevent tooth decay and keep your gums healthy. That's because of its antiseptic qualities. So if you want the 'herbal' way to do it, stock up on the tincture.

CANKER SORES: Traditionally, myrrh was used by the early American settlers to treat canker sores – painful dry ulcers that form in the mouth. In fact, I think you can bet that if the treatment was introduced to America by those settlers, it must have originated somewhere else. To treat a canker sore simply open up a tablet of powdered myrrh and dab it on the sore, repeating as often as necessary.

A WORD OF CAUTION: Please refer to the dosage instructions and take accordingly.

INTERESTING FACTS: Ancient Egyptians added the gum resin from myrrh to insect repellents. It was also traditionally used in embalming and for incense in temples.

Nettle

Despite its prickly content, nettle is a kind plant, great for healing many ailments and one that has done so for hundreds of years. It's also very readily available – just check out your average hedgerow for a start! Fortunately, when it's boiled, the bristles disappear, so the only problem is gathering it, and if you wear gloves this shouldn't be too difficult. Or you can buy nettle teas, juices and extracts – whatever. All parts of the plant are used and each is good for different things. So if you're thinking of it as a treatment, then make sure you've got the right part, so to speak.

ARTHRITIS: Nettle leaf extract is a Native American remedy for rheumatic pains, and studies have shown that taking it along with a particular prescription drug allowed sufferers to reduce their dosage of the drug. So it can't be bad! If you are a sufferer you could always try a cup of nettle tea a day. There are those who actually deliberately hit themselves with nettles, when their joints get sore. Rather you than me, is all I can say!

URINARY TRACT INFECTIONS: Again, nettle leaf tea can help fight infection by flushing out bacteria. Drink several cups of tea a day until it clears, or try incorporating it into your diet, perhaps just by taking one cup a day, if you're a regular sufferer. To make the tea you can pour hot (not boiling) water over one teaspoon of dried leaf, steep for five minutes, then strain. If you drink a lot of nettle tea, however, do remember that it is a diuretic and you should make sure you drink lots of other fluids, so you don't become dehydrated.

HAYFEVER: While it might seem strange to recommend a plant to cure a condition which is often triggered by a proximity to plants, nettle leaf tea or extract might help minimise the unpleasant symptoms of hayfever. In this case you might be better buying capsules and taking them according to the instructions.

ENLARGED PROSTATE: Studies indicate that nettle root can be helpful in slowing the development of this condition, although the actual reasons for it are unclear. If it's something you're worried about at all, or think you might have early signs of then you could try taking capsules. Just make sure they are from the root not the leaves of the plant. If symptoms persist you should consult your doctor.

A WORD OF CAUTION: Apart from the obvious point I've already mentioned with regard to picking nettles, nettle is quite safe, although it can sometimes cause indigestion. You should, however, avoid nettle if you are pregnant or breast feeding. If you are diabetic, or taking blood thinning or blood pressure drugs, you should consult your doctor first. Also, remember that if you are taking any prescription drugs for the conditions listed above, you should speak to your doctor first. Don't stop taking prescribed drugs without your doctor's say so.

INTERESTING FACTS: Nettle was used by the Ancient Greeks to treat coughs. The fibres from the stem were traditionally used to make cloth. The leaves were eaten in some cultures to promote hair and nail growth. The Latin name Urtico Dioica means 'I burn'. Not a bad description of what you will do if you touch it!

Omega-3 fatty acids

While this might sound like the latest group to top the charts, omega-3 fatty acids have much more to do with food. For the uninitiated they are in fact fish oils, mostly found in cold water fish. Tuna, salmon and mackerel are excellent sources. But leafy green vegetables, and certain vegetable oils, also contain them. If you eat a lot of fish and leafy greens, then fine, you're certainly doing your bit towards keeping yourself healthy and hopefully reducing your risk of certain conditions. Because that's where the omega-3s come into their own. If you don't like fish or can't eat it, and you don't like leafy greens, then perhaps you should take a look at what omega-3 can do and hopefully think again.

HEART DISEASE: Studies now demonstrate that, contrary to their name, omega-3 fatties, aren't 'fat' at all. What they do is protect the heart by mopping up the nasties that gather 'on the pipes'. If you want to improve your quality of life, if you have heart disease, or want to take some preventative measures, it's not all down to exercise. It's also down to eating wisely. So think about increasing your fish and leafy green intake. And as I've said before, that doesn't mean eating all kinds of boring dishes. It also doesn't mean visiting the chipper every night either, by the way. Fish can be done in a variety of sauces and tuna lends itself to pasta dishes, baked potatoes and salads. So think again. The health benefits are enormous.

CANCER PREVENTION: Okay, the sad fact is that cancer can strike the healthiest individual. However, some preliminary research suggests that omega-3 fatty acids may help keep breast tissue healthy and have a role to play in preventing colon cancer. Remember, we are what we eat. The cancer and heart disease rates in the UK are high. Much of that is down to diet, our preference for stodgy pies and convenient, processed food – with no vegetables at all in many instances. By the way, there's absolutely nothing wrong with eating stodgy pies and processed foods, I'm personally rather fond of them! But we need to balance that more with nutritious things.

INFLAMMATORY BOWEL DISEASE: Again, there are studies to show that people taking three grams of fish oil a day, stayed symptom free. If you're a sufferer, examine your diet. Do you eat lots of fish? If not, how about making a start?

MENSTRUAL CRAMPS: In some instances, omega-3 can help this condition because it reduces inflammation. It might be a good idea to look at your diet around the time your period starts and eat lots of fish.

RHEUMATOID ARTHRITIS: I've talked about this earlier and how it destroys the joints. Well, there is some research that suggests omega-3 fatty acid helps reduce the inflammation and stiffness of this condition.

HIV INFECTION: I'm not about to say that omega-3 can cure this.

Simply that there is evidence to suggest that nutrition can boost the immune system and that if sufferers take plenty of fruit and vegetables in their diet they may take longer to develop full-blown AIDS. In some instances, adding omega-3 doubled life expectancy.

A WORD OF CAUTION: So far I haven't come across any.

INTERESTING FACT: Saturated fat is a major cause of heart disease.

Onion

If you include lots of onion in your diet, then good. If you don't, then think about it. Onions contain many compounds as well as antiseptic qualities, which make them useful healers. They're very good for you, too. From pizza toppings to soup, to putting them in the casserole, there are so many ways to eat them. But using them as a poultice can also be beneficial, as you will see below, and if they're things you have in the cupboard anyway, you could save yourself a fortune in the herbal remedies stakes!

BURNS: A good onion paste can treat a burn. Just mash or puree and put the resulting paste on the damaged area. The antiseptic in onion will soon start work to soothe and heal the burn. A good tip is to include the onion skin in this as it is especially good at reducing inflammation.

ASTHMA: Onion isn't maybe the most effective method of treating asthma, but if you're a sufferer then make sure there are lots in your diet. Onion does contain anti-asthmatic compounds.

INSECT BITES: Because onion also contains quercetin – an anti-inflammatory compound – it could help take the sting out of insect bites. Make a poultice as suggested above (see Burns).

SCABIES: Soothe away scabies and other itchy skin problems by boiling onion skins in a pot of water for 15 minutes. When it's cool, apply it to the affected area. The quercetin in onion is what does the trick.

VARICOSE VEINS: Eating plenty onions and thus increasing the body's quercetin supply may well help sufferers of this condition. You can also try making a poultice or onion wash with the skins, as suggested above and applying to the swollen veins.

PNEUMONIA: Let's not kid ourselves, onions won't treat pneumonia single-handedly, but they are very good for respiratory complaints from colds to flu. Tempt sufferers with onion soup, or add plenty to a good lentil or chicken recipe. It can't do any harm and will probably do a lot of good.

A WORD OF CAUTION: None that I can think of, unless you have some kind of food allergy to onions. They're safe, easily obtainable and can even be home-grown. I know a few who find onions 'repeat' and cause fairly severe indigestion. I personally love them.

INTERESTING FACTS: Onions have been cultivated from time immemorial. It is one of the earliest cultivated plants. One variety in ancient Egypt was even accorded divine honours and represented on monuments!

Oregano

Oregano is a member of the mint family. A rather pleasant herb I like as a food flavouring, especially in lentil soup, or on pasta. It contains antioxidant properties, ones that protect cells from damage. In particular, it is good for reducing inflammation. If you suffer from the following, then you should certainly think about including it in your diet, as I do, on a regular basis.

ARTHRITIS: Since arthritis is joint inflammation, oregano can help keep it a bay a little. If you are a sufferer you might want to do more than just add it to your food, you might want to try herbal medicines that contain it. Health stores and supermarkets both have herbal remedies for arthritis, in capsule or tincture form, which you can take according to the instructions. Make sure oregano is included in the formula. Ask at your health store for teas containing oregano, or add half a teaspoon of dried herb to a cup of boiling water, strain and drink.

ASTHMA: Since oregano contains anti-asthmatic qualities, adding it to your diet might help improve this condition. It can certainly do no harm. You can also ask at your health store for products containing it, which can be taken on a regular basis, such as tea or tincture.

EMPHYSEMA: Oregano is an expectorant. While it won't cure this condition, adding it you your diet generally could help improve it. Or try putting a spoonful in a basin of hot water, placing a towel over your head and inhaling the vapour.

SINUSITIS: Use the herb as directed above to inhale the vapour, or drink lots of oregano tea – ask at your health store, or make your own – to help ease congestion and thus soothe this condition.

A WORD OF CAUTION: None that I know of. Oregano is safe and delicious, but always follow instructions.

INTERESTING FACT: Oregano is mainly used in Italian cuisine. Don't look to buy oregano plants as such. If you want to plant it, look for marjoram.

Osteopathy

WHAT IS IT? This is another therapy the Americans can claim as one of 'theirs', so to speak, although its actual basis is not so different from some other therapies. Osteopaths believe that all the systems of the body are linked. If one is out of kilter, then it affects the others. So they focus their attention on the bones and muscles to find the problem.

HOW DOES IT WORK? Well, if I told you about the agonising session I once endured many years ago you might not go at all! Although the problem was solved! Things have changed quite a bit since then, I gather. Nowadays if you go to an osteopath they will want to know all about your illness, your emotional health, lifestyle and possibly even your diet, to see if that also needs correcting. They will check over your spine, muscles and joints, and manipulate where necessary to correct any problem and promote healing, apparently – and I quote – 'with painless thrusts'.

WHAT DOES IT HELP IN PARTICULAR? This treatment is very good for back and neck pain, headaches, knee and joint injuries. It can also relax muscles and help with stress and poor circulation, improve posture and increase mobility. 'Painless thrusts' apart, I certainly had no more back trouble after visiting an osteopath and, accordingly, I swear by them.

HOW LONG SHOULD A COURSE OF TREATMENT LAST? A first session may last an hour and if you need to go back, then this is generally shorter, perhaps 20 minutes or so. The amount of sessions you need depends on the problem and how beneficial the visit was. Often one will do the trick.

HOW DO I GO ABOUT GETTING THIS TREATMENT? Osteopaths have been around a long time. Even in Britain! Some even advertise in the Yellow Pages and are attached to hospitals. Your health shop or centre are also good places to start.

A WORD OF CAUTION: Make sure the osteopath you choose is properly qualified. Sometimes the best recommendations come by word of mouth. Although osteopathy treats conditions of the joints and bones, if you actually have a broken bone, severe joint inflammation, bone cancer, a prolapsed disc or have had a spinal fusion, this isn't for you.

INTERESTING FACT: Osteopathy was founded by a Missouri surgeon after losing three of his children to spinal meningitis.

Parsley

Parsley's a lovely little herb. One we tend to use to garnish food rather than actually eat. Yet it has so many uses, it's a shame to do this. Start sprinkling it into your cooking, instead of just popping a drop on top of the soup for serving, or sticking round the plate when you do a buffet. You'll be amazed at the things it is good for.

In addition to everything else, it's also a very high source of fluorine, a bone strengthener. So if you're worried about keeping those bones healthy, adding parsley to your diet is a good way to do it!

BLADDER INFECTIONS: Parsley was traditionally used to treat bladder infections. It's an excellent diuretic that flushes the bacteria off the bladder walls. You can try making a tea by steeping the leaves for 15 minutes in a cup of water, staining then drinking. Or eat some sprigs. Including it regularly in your diet can help keep these infections down generally.

BRUISES: Rubbing parsley leaves on a bruise can clear it up within a day or two. You would, of course, have to do this more than once. If you have a plant in your garden you'll know what to do the next time you've got one.

LOSS OF LIBIDO (WOMEN): Sorry you men, but some things are for women only and we are covering your conditions where appropriate! But for women readers, if you've lost the interest lately and really can't be bothered, but wish you could do something about it, then try parsley. This little herb has a long history of helping with just this problem! Traditionally, it was used for all women-related troubles, childbirth, breast-feeding, bringing on menstruation and also for increasing desire! You might have to eat lots, but so what! Seriously, add it to your diet regularly as well as trying the other remedies mentioned (see Libido loss, page 79) and good luck!

BREAST-FEEDING: As mentioned above, parsley is particularly good for women. You could almost call it 'The Woman's Herb'. If you are breast-feeding, it can reduce the tenderness, especially if the tenderness is down to fluid retention. It is also very good when you are thinking about weaning the baby, since it helps reduce the milk. Buy some fresh leaves and eat them in a salad, or grow your own.

HALITOSIS: Banish bad breath by taking a sprig of parsley after your meal, or keeping the parsley till last. (See Halitosis, page 62.)

A WORD OF CAUTION: None I can think of. Parsley is very easy to find, dried or fresh and can be grown in your garden or window box.

INTERESTING FACT: Parsley is one of the Scarborough Fair herbs, mentioned in the song. In cooking it works very well with sage, rosemary and thyme.

Peppermint

Peppermint is another of those wonderful herbs that do so much. It has been commercially grown for years, but mainly as a food flavouring. Let's face it, we all love a box of chocolate mints. It's also used in toothpastes – at least the flavouring is. But peppermint has so many other uses, you'd be surprised. I know I was when I first started recommending it!

HALITOSIS: Peppermint can definitely help with this problem. But use the tea to gargle with. Often toothpastes only contain the flavouring. (See Halitosis, page 62.)

SCABIES: One thing I have discovered is that peppermint is a very good antiseptic. If you suffer from this irritating condition you can certainly try using it. Either make a tea with peppermint leaves, and when it is cool, strain and apply it to the affected skin, or run a bath and pour the tea in.

NAUSEA: I always keep a stash of peppermint tea bags handy in case anyone doesn't feel too well. I know I could make my own but I don't always have time. What I like best about peppermint tea is that it can stop people retching and help settle the digestive system down.

MORNING SICKNESS: I wouldn't, however, recommend it if you're pregnant. In large amounts it can sometimes cause miscarriage. You could, though, try chewing on a candied stick. (See Morning sickness, page 90.)

HEARTBURN: If you suffer from heartburn then you can certainly try some peppermint tea. Mint generally eases the digestion. Even if it's just the flavouring, I find even just sucking a peppermint sweet slowly can soon ease this problem.

HEADACHE: Although lavender is traditionally associated with easing headaches, peppermint can also help. I don't know if it's the smell that does it. In this instance you would have to try using peppermint oil, however, which you should be able to get in a health shop. Mix it with lavender and rub on the temples. Don't try to take the oil. It's very toxic.

FEVER: Peppermint's cooling qualities can help reduce a fever. Try a cup of peppermint tea if you've got one.

GINGIVITIS: In addition to freshening the breath, peppermint tea can help gingivitis. Because it contains antiseptic qualities, it keeps the mouth generally healthy. Rather than drinking the tea you can try using it as a mouthwash and if you have the plant in your garden, you can brew your own!

SINUSITIS: Either rub some peppermint oil on your temples, or add some to your steamy bath water if you've got this condition. I think I'm right in saying that the vapours will help clear the sinuses generally. Just don't drink the oil. If you don't have any oil then use some fresh leaves in hot water, or inhale the vapours from a cup of tea. In some cultures, people actually stick peppermint leaves up their noses to relieve symptoms. I wouldn't recommend this, but inhaling the vapours should certainly help.

EMPHYSEMA: As well as sinusitis, I sometimes recommend peppermint tea or inhaling the vapours of the oil, to help with this condition. The menthol is very good for thinning mucus. Peppermint also comes in capsule form, which might be something you could look into, if you suffer from this condition. Ask at your health shop.

A WORD OF CAUTION: As I say above, please don't drink peppermint tea if you're pregnant – find something else. In some instances peppermint can actually aggravate heartburn. So if you find it makes things worse not better, then stop taking it. Otherwise, peppermint is very good to use.

INTERESTING FACT: The Romans, who certainly knew how to eat, chewed mint sprigs after meals in order to soothe the digestion. And no wonder! Some meals went on for days!

Potassium

Potassium is usually so plentiful in the human body that most people have more than enough in their food and don't need to take supplements. This is good because potassium works pretty hard. One of the things it does is covert blood sugar into energy and release it when needed. Fruit, vegetables and orange juice are all excellent sources of potassium but many other foodstuffs have it as well. Yoghurt and avocados are also good sources. Making sure you eat lots of potatoes and bananas can apparently decrease your risk of having a stroke – according to certain studies, anyway. It can also help prevent kidney stones.

REDUCING HIGH BLOOD PRESSURE: People who regularly eat high potassium diets have much lower blood pressure than those who don't. The reductions are greatest where people already have high blood pressure. It makes sense, therefore, if you have this problem to take a look at your diet and think seriously about incorporating into it the things I've mentioned above. Supplements can be taken but, as you will see from the word of caution, it's much simpler to increase your intake through foods.

A WORD OF CAUTION: Because potassium supplements can cause an upset stomach they must always be taken with food. If you suffer from a kidney disorder, or take medication to control high blood pressure or heart disease, you mustn't take supplements without medical supervision. The food is fine, but not the supplements. That's why I'm saying get what you can through your diet. If you're taking diuretic drugs, digitalis, beta-blockers, anti-inflammatories or medication for angina, you can't even take them with medical supervision. That's because they can sort of undo each other and develop a condition called hypokalaemia, which isn't a Greek word for good morning, but a nasty muscle twitching thing you really wouldn't want.

INTERESTING FACT: Potassium imbalances generally correct themselves.

Psyllium

This strange-sounding plant – a sort of 'silly him' – isn't as daft as you might think. It's a species of plantain, from a group of plants we, in the UK, think of as weeds – though our Asian and Mediterranean counterparts grow it commercially because of its laxative benefits. The seeds have husks which swell when soaked in water, giving the bowel plenty of bulk and fibre to work on. If these things are a problem for you, then you could consider adding some to your diet, although I'd like you to read on before doing so. If you're interested you can ask at your health shop for preparations and see how you get on. It might just be the remedy you've been looking for!

CONSTIPATION: Taking three to ten tablespoons of seeds a day can help chronic constipation. That's according to the German Commission E who examine such things. It sounds a lot, I know. What you might be best to do is find how many work for you. A more typical dose might be to take up to six 660 mg capsules a day, drinking a full glass of water with each dose, or stirring either one teaspoon of husks or two teaspoons of powdered seed in a large glass of water and drinking after meals. You'll note I'm hammering away at the water. That's because they need lots of water to work, otherwise they can swell and obstruct the digestive tract.

DIARRHOEA: Conversely psyllium also works by stopping diarrhoea. How? Well, you just don't drink so much water.

INFLAMMATORY BOWEL DISEASE: IBD is no joke if you have it. Chronic diarrhoea is one of the symptoms. Taking psyllium seeds could help.

HAEMORRHOIDS: Psyllium can help relieve the symptoms associated with this condition. Follow the instructions above for constipation.

IRRITABLE BOWEL SYNDROME (IBS): Because they keep the bowels moving regularly, relieving constipation and bloating, the seeds can help this condition.

A WORD OF CAUTION: If you have asthma, don't take this herb. It can trigger allergic reactions. If this happens, discontinue use. It can also be dangerous if the intestine is obstructed. So if you're suddenly suffering chronic constipation, with no clear idea why, consult your doctor. Also, don't take psyllium if you're diabetic. Some preparations of it contain sugar.

INTERESTING FACT: The seeds have been used for hundreds of years in Europe to cure constipation.

Quercetin

This little-known supplement, or to give it it's proper title, flavonoid (meaning plant tint or pigment), has some wonderful advantages, especially to me and others like me who suffer from asthma. The phrase 'an apple a day keeps the doctor away' may well stem from this very supplement, as the main source of quercetin is found in apples and also in onions. Quercetin mainly acts, or let's say acts better, when combined with other members of the flavonoid family.

ASTHMA: As it reduces inflammation in the airways, quercetin is useful for asthma sufferers. It can also prevent allergic reactions to pollen and is therefore a great antihistamine. It is said to keep the lungs clear and all essential passageways open.

CATARACT: Some studies show that quercetin prevents the build up of a type of sugar known medically as sorbitol and can therefore prevent, or at least slow down, cataract formation.

DIABETES: Again, due to quercetin's apparent ability to combat, or at least reduce, the rate of sorbitol build up, it is thought diabetics could also benefit from its use.

GOUT: Working on the same theory, quercetin's ability to reduce inflammation may go some way to preventing this acutely painful disease.

A WORD OF CAUTION: Actually, there doesn't appear to be any! Although quercetin can be administered in supplement form, it is recommended that the best and most effective intake, should be in our food – apples in particular.

INTERESTING FACTS: I found quite a few whilst doing my studies – some I must admit I am slightly wary of, however. Studies have shown that those who take high dosages of quercetin are less likely to contract, or are better able to combat, many illnesses, including some of the very serious ones, such as cancer of the lungs, breast and stomach. The general opinion here is that the risk is greatly reduced if a high intake of dietary quercetin is taken.

I was told whilst researching that many years ago quercetin was found to bring on cancer in animals. However, later tests dismissed this. Further research has shown that those who eat foods containing quercetin are, in fact, more likely to avoid contracting cancer.

It has to be said, however, that a great many of the recent studies remain controversial, with one group categorically saying yes, quercetin can reduce the risk of cancer, while other groups state that they find no such connection. However, the overall opinion remains that it may well be a preventative measure.

Red Pepper (cayenne powder)

Red pepper is good for so many things, it's not possible to overlook them here.

HEART DISEASE: Like garlic, onions and ginger, red pepper contains compounds that help thin the blood, making it less likely to clot and in turn reducing the risk of heart attack. Think about including it in your diet on a regular basis. It's so easy just to add to your food when you are preparing it.

ARTHRITIS: Like stinging nettle, red pepper may cause quite a bit of pain when applied to the body – in this case, the tongue – but often pain meets pain and the problem is solved. Well, sort of. Nothing's ever so easy, is it! Please don't even think of putting it on your tongue, by the way. What you can try, however, is adding it to your cooking. It does have a chemical that helps the body fight pain, especially arthritic pain. So, if you are a sufferer, then diet can help! You can also try applying it to the skin – as a cream, of course. Look for ones containing capsaicin at your health shop. Then apply it to the affected areas.

BUNIONS: The same goes for this condition. Try to find a cream containing capsaicin or cut open a red pepper and put it on your bunion if it's sore.

DRY MOUTH: Contrary to what you might expect, putting red pepper in your food can actually alleviate this condition. That's because capsaicin gets the salivary gland going.

FEVER: Adding red pepper to your food can help reduce a fever. If you have a bad cold, you know what they say about feeding it! Well, this is definitely fever food!

HEADACHE: Because red pepper has pain-relieving compounds it is good for getting rid of a headache. More importantly, where cluster types are concerned, red pepper has been actively shown to prevent them. Since these are so debilitating, I don't just recommend putting red pepper on your food, however, I'd actually recommend taking cayenne capsules. Ask at your health shop and take according to the instructions.

SHINGLES: Red pepper is good for easing this painful condition – one that can continue to cause pain in the nerves long after the actual ailment has gone. Either ask at your health shop for a cream containing capsaicin or add red pepper to a skin lotion and put it on.

PSORIASIS: The same as the above goes for this condition.

A WORD OF CAUTION: If you are using a cream containing capsaicin, be sure to wash your hands afterwards. Do not rub this cream into your eyes, as this can cause irritation. If you find you are allergic to products containing red pepper or its compounds, discontinue use.

INTERESTING FACT: Red pepper is also good for toothache, indigestion, backache, emphysema and weight control!

Reflexology

WHAT IS IT? The precise origins of reflexology are unclear, but it is based on the belief that the feet have a lot to answer for! While *we* might see the soles of our feet as an area of calloused skin and corns, reflexologists see a coded map of the entire body. The toes correspond to the head and neck, the balls of the feet reflect the heart and so on, while the points on the feet relate to the points of the body. And you thought they were just for standing on!

HOW DOES IT WORK? This isn't actually terribly clear, although it is thought that when pressure is applied to the feet, the body's natural painkillers are released. And before you say, 'I'm on mine all day,' that doesn't help I'm afraid. In reflexology, the feet are rubbed, and then the practitioner concentrates on the tense areas. Any discomfort you feel should ease. As each particular area is pressed, you should feel a tingling in the part of the body that it corresponds with.

WHAT DOES IT HELP IN PARTICULAR? If you suffer from stress, anxiety, digestive problems and headaches, you might find reflexology helpful. It can also benefit sufferers from sciatica, arthritis, acne and other skin conditions, insomnia, PMT, asthma and irritable bowel syndrome.

HOW LONG SHOULD A COURSE OF TREATMENT LAST? Like everything else this depends upon the condition. But treatments are usually given on a weekly basis to begin with and last between 30 and 60 minutes. Then they just take place when appropriate. If you can learn where the points for your condition are you can perform reflexology on yourself.

HOW DO I GO ABOUT GETTING THIS TREATMENT? Many people who practice massage and chiropody are also trained in reflexology. Ask at your health centre or shop for the name of a reflexologist who is available locally.

A WORD OF CAUTION: Like so many other therapies, reflexology will not cure your condition. So don't dance along to a therapist thinking, 'This is it!' It's not. Reflexology is helpful for existing conditions, often in relieving the pain and stress associated with them. Also, remember that reflexologists are not qualified to diagnose disease, so if there's something troubling you, see a doctor. And if you have serious circulatory problems, blood clots, thrombosis or a foot injury, talk to your doctor first before going off to see a reflexologist. Tell your reflexologist if you are pregnant, have gallstones, kidney stones, or a pacemaker.

INTERESTING FACT: Present day reflexology was developed in the early 1900s by a nose and throat specialist and refined in the 1930s more or less to how we know it today.

Reiki

WHAT IS IT? Well, first of all, Reiki is pronounced 'ray kee' if you want to go asking about it, and it is another ancient therapy – one in which healing energy is actually channelled through a practitioner's hands into the person receiving treatment.

HOW DOES IT WORK? Like many other therapies, Reiki concentrates on achieving mind and body unity, thus helping the body to heal itself. The practitioner's intention in laying on his or her hands is not to heal, however, but to break up blockages so that the healing energy can flow more freely. Although this sounds intense, Reiki is actually so gentle that many people fall asleep in sessions. That's because Reiki generally begins with a quiet period of contemplation and involves doing nothing more strenuous than lying on a padded massage table. For you that is. The practitioner will scan your body for blockages and some can simply tell where the blockage is by noting if their hands are hot. Then they will touch various places systematically to channel the healing energy.

WHAT DOES IT HELP IN PARTICULAR? While it cannot heal these conditions, Reiki has been shown to help relieve the pain of arthritis and multiple sclerosis. It also helps with depression, stress and the emotional problems associated with certain terminal conditions.

HOW LONG SHOULD A COURSE OF TREATMENT LAST? An actual session lasts between 60 and 90 minutes. The number of sessions you have depends on the condition. Chronic conditions often require long-term treatment.

HOW DO I GO ABOUT GETTING THIS TREATMENT? Ask your doctor or at your health shop if they know of any practitioners locally. Some people who practice Reiki are often already trained in massage or physical therapy and have added Reiki as another string to their bow, so to speak, by taking training.

A WORD OF CAUTION: While it has been shown that Reiki can help certain conditions, it is not a substitute for medical care. As a therapy it is there to support ongoing treatment. Just because it releases healing powers, don't expect it to 'mend' conditions.

INTERESTING FACT: Reiki is thought to have originated in Tibet. It was then brought to Japan in the early 1900s.

Riboflavin

Also known as vitamin B2, riboflavin plays an important part in converting protein, fats and carbohydrates into the energy we need to grow and develop properly. In addition, the body uses extra riboflavin to keep tissue in good repair and speed the healing of wounds, burns and other injuries, so it's fairly vital that we have enough. Many scientists think we haven't looked hard enough at the role it could play in treating conditions that affect the nervous system.

ALZHEIMER'S, FATIGUE AND STRESS: Interestingly, the elderly are often deficient in riboflavin, so are alcoholics. The signs of too little riboflavin are cracking of the lips at the corners of the mouth, flaky skin around the nose and ear lobes, and itchy eyes. A low red blood count is another sign.

MIGRAINES: Because many migraine sufferers have low reserves of energy in their brain, scientists think that taking riboflavin could help. One of the things it does is boost energy levels throughout the body generally. A recent European study has shown that those taking riboflavin suffered from fewer migraines, although the severity and duration of the migraines that did occur were not lessened. Riboflavin, however, has fewer side effects than many prescription drugs. For prevention you would need to take 400 mg every morning. And please note the word 'prevention'. Riboflavin does not treat a migraine once it is there.

FATIGUE: If you are constantly tired, it may be that your red blood cell count is low and needs boosting. You could try taking daily supplements till your tiredness disappears.

SKIN PROBLEMS: Many people with skin blemishes and various skin conditions have a riboflavin deficiency. Again, taking a small supplement – 50 mg a day – could improve the look of your skin.

A WORD OF CAUTION: Do not take riboflavin with alcohol as this can interfere with the digestive tract's ability to absorb it. Also, if you use oral contraceptives or psychiatric drugs, check with your doctor first as dosage requirements would need to be adjusted. Apart from that, riboflavin is easy and safe to take. In addition to being available as a single supplement from health stores, it is often contained in multivitamin products.

INTERESTING FACT: Riboflavin was originally discovered in 1879 but no one knew what it was or what it could do for another 50 years.

Rosemary

A plant of the mint family, rosemary was not only widely used by ancient civilisations, but highly esteemed by them as well. Its aromatic qualities and medicinal qualities were prized. Both in literature and folklore, it was called the herb of remembrance. But in modern times it has fallen out of favour somewhat, coming to be valued for its perfume, or for chucking on the lamb roast of a Sunday afternoon. If you do the latter, then good. As I always say, every little helps. But rosemary has other uses, too. Here are some of them.

ARTHRITIS: Rosemary contains antioxidants which help to prevent the body cells ageing. Therefore it might help slow arthritis. In addition to putting it in your food, you can try wearing perfumes containing rosemary oil, looking for bath products that do, or following our instructions below (in Pain).

ALZHEIMER'S DISEASE: Because rosemary helps slow ageing generally, it could be of help in preventing this condition or slowing the progress of it. (See Alzheimer's disease, page 13.)

FAINTING: The oil that gives rosemary its aroma is full of cineole. This is active when inhaled, ingested, or applied to the skin. So if someone faints and you have rosemary oil, or a perfume containing rosemary, pop a drop or two on a tissue under their nose. A cup of rosemary tea can also help revive the spirits of someone who has fainted and get them back on their feet. Use a spoonful of dried herb in a cup of boiling water, strain then sweeten, if you don't have any herbal tea bags containing it.

WRINKLES: Used regularly in cooking or made into a tea (see above) rosemary could help skin keep its elasticity. So chucking it on the lamb isn't such a bad idea.

PAIN: A rosemary bath can not only help soothe painful joints but it may also relax you generally. Either look for bath products containing rosemary, or put some dried rosemary in a cheesecloth bag and run the water over it.

AVAILABILITY: Rosemary is easily obtainable in herb form. Most supermarkets stock it. You can also ask at you local health shop about other products containing it, such as herbal tea, and look at the various ranges of bath and body products that exist. From deodorant to shampoo, more and more companies are going in for a natural range, with all sorts of benefits for our health.

A WORD OF CAUTION: Some reports show that during pregnancy, the intake of rosemary may harm the unborn foetus.

INTERESTING FACT: The inclusion of rosemary in the words of the old song 'Scarborough Fair' shows how highly the plant was previously regarded. In addition to putting rosemary on your lamb, sprinkle on some sage and thyme. Then when it is cooked, put half a teaspoon of each into your gravy, with a scoosh of tomato puree, pour on the lamb and reheat for 20 minutes. The result is absolutely delicious.

Sage

Personally sage is one of my favourite herbs. Even the name implies what it can do and what a clever little herb it is. It's also fabulous for flavouring a Sunday roast, which is my favourite way to take it (see Rosemary, above). Like many other herbs down the years, some of its uses have been forgotten. For centuries it was highly regarded as being useful for preventing ageing and strengthening the memory. Even the Romans swore by it. The Victorians, too, had many 'folklore' uses for it. Let's take a look at some. They certainly are surprising!

ALZHEIMER'S DISEASE: Because sage is full of antioxidants, using it regularly in food or as a tea, might help prevent this disease occurring. (See Alzheimer's disease, page 13.)

GINGIVITIS: The Victorians recommended rubbing sage leaves on your teeth to get rid of stains. So if you can't move the brown marks, you could try buying a sage plant for your garden. Then there's gingivitis – redness, swelling and bleeding of the gums, in other words – using sage leaves in this way may also help prevent that developing.

TONSILLITIS: The Germans recommend gargling with hot sage. So perhaps if you have tonsillitis you can either try taking a herbal tea with sage in it, or perhaps preparing your own gargle, by pouring boiling water on a spoonful of dried sage. Strain, allow to cool and gargle the results.

WRINKLES: Since sage's wonderful properties seem to keep those who take it feeling young, you might find it helps the skin do the same. So include it generally in your diet. The Victorians also thought that sage tea kept the hair from going white. Must try some! You never know!

CRAMP: Another favourite use of sage amongst the Victorians was hot sage baths, for the soothing of sore limbs and for cramp sufferers. You can try putting a sage tea bag in the hot water, or putting some dried sage or sage leaves in a cheesecloth bag and running the water through it.

YEAST INFECTIONS: Sage tea or a sage bath (see above) might help soothe candida infections.

ASTHMA: Some of the compounds in sage might help sufferers, although perhaps sage isn't so effective here. However, you could try putting some sage in a basin of hot water, placing a towel over your head and inhaling.

AVAILABILITY: Sage is very easy to find. The herb can be bought dried in most supermarkets. You can ask at your health shop for preparations containing sage, try making your own tea by boiling the leaves with hot water and straining, or, best of all, grow your own. Then you will have all the sage you need.

A WORD OF CAUTION: In very high doses sage can occasionally cause convulsions. So do as the name implies and be wise.

INTERESTING FACTS: According to the Romans: 'Why should a wise man die while there is sage in his garden?' And the olde English: 'He who would live for aye, must eat sage all through May.'

Shiatsu

WHAT IS IT? As its name suggests, Shiatsu hails from Japan. The word translates as 'finger pressure' and yes, that's what it is, up to a point. But practitioners of this aged and venerable therapy also use their palms, elbows, knees and feet – ouch! – to apply pressure to points along the body's energy channels, thus ensuring that everything flows freely. Sounds painful, I know. In many ways it is similar to acupressure.

HOW DOES IT WORK? Well, before you go getting the idea that it's a bit like trampling grapes, I should add that there are many different types of Shiatsu massage. Some practitioners press, hold, stretch and rotate parts of the body. Others use their bodies to apply strong pressure. And yes, some do use their feet. On the whole, however, the treatment is relaxing and is aimed at relieving the tension that has built up in the body, thus releasing the natural painkillers we all have in our systems.

WHAT DOES IT HELP IN PARTICULAR? Like certain other treatments and therapies, Shiatsu is best used to prevent illness and keep the body healthy. Sufferers from headaches, insomnia, muscle and menstrual cramps have reported improvements to these conditions, however. So have those with shoulder and neck pain and arthritis. In some instances, too, it has been known to help people suffering asthma and constipation.

HOW LONG SHOULD A COURSE OF TREATMENT LAST? Actual sessions last from 45 minutes to an hour and it can take four to eight sessions to resolve certain problems. Long-term or chronic conditions – i.e. things you've suffered from for months – may need more sessions. Also, when you first go for treatment, the practitioner will spend some time asking you about your lifestyle and diet as well as your medical history.

HOW DO I GO ABOUT GETTING THIS TREATMENT? If you are thinking about trying this treatment then make sure whoever you choose is registered and that they are someone you feel comfortable with. Often a recommendation from a friend or health shop is the place to start. Nowadays many therapy practitioners leave their card with health shops, so you can ask there.

A WORD OF CAUTION: Shiatsu involves a lot of touching, so if you're not a touchy-feely kind of person, then this might not be the treatment for you. You should also avoid this therapy if you have varicose veins, phlebitis or any circulatory ailment, or if you have had recent surgery, a fracture or sprain – obviously! – radiation therapy or chemotherapy. If you have a rash or infectious skin disease, Shiatsu is not for you and massage should be avoided in any area where a tumour is cited, or on your stomach if you are in the first three months of pregnancy, have a hernia, have any kind of abdominal pain or have eaten within the last two hours.

INTERESTING FACT: The business of using massage to help keep people healthy goes back to ancient China. But as time passed, the health benefit side of things was dropped and massage was used mainly for pleasure and relaxation. It's only in the last century that things have turned round again for this ancient therapy and its medical benefits have again become clear.

Soy bean

For hundreds of years soya has been the staple diet in many Asian countries and it's easy to see why. Not only is it low in fat, as well as being cholesterol free – something that's ideal if this is a problem for you – it contains compounds that boost the immune system. It can also provide the body with amino acids, which makes it a favourite of vegetarians. Pretty good I'd say and if you're worried about certain other effects to do with beans generally, which I won't mention here, yes, we have a section on that too (see page 50)!

MENOPAUSE: Studies show that soy beans can help stop hot flushes and regulate hormones in menopausal women. This is because they contain substances that help replace the oestrogen. So if you suffer hot flushes and want to give soy beans a go, then you might find it actually improves this condition.

OSTEOPOROSIS: Although the link between soy beans and osteoporosis is still being researched, it is generally thought that soy beans contain compounds that increase bone density, thus helping prevent this painful condition. If it's one you're worried about, then add soy beans to your diet.

VAGINITIS: Soya does help stop the dryness and irritation associated with the menopause so it is possible that eating soy beans regularly may help long-term sufferers of this condition.

A WORD OF CAUTION: Although cooked soy beans are safe to eat, some people are allergic and should therefore avoid soya products. In some cases, too, soy beans can interfere with mineral absorption. So, if you are taking mineral extracts, this is something to consider. Otherwise, they can certainly be helpful and healthy things to eat as well as being easily available in supermarkets.

INTERESTING FACT: Asian women have a lower incidence of breast cancer.

Spinach

Well we've all heard of Popeye and obviously seen what the average helping of spinach can do for him. In cartoon terms maybe! A sort of graphic equivalent of 'in your dreams'. This vegetable is, however, a good mineral source. A bit strange to look at maybe, and not always to everyone's taste when it comes to eating it. Popeye was obviously made of tough stuff. You can, however, take it in other ways than boiled. Putting it in soup with cabbage and asparagus is one way. Or in a flan. It's a good food to eat if you're pregnant. Not only does it help keep you healthy but the baby too. Saying you should eat it if you're a vegetarian is probably a bit like telling your granny to suck eggs, but I'm going to anyway. Spinach is high in zinc, a mineral we all require and one most non-vegetarians get from meat. So it makes sense if you're cutting meat out to replace it with this. Because of the things it contains, spinach is good for:

PREVENTING STROKE: That's because of the amount of folate in it, a substance that helps stop the arteries narrowing and one, incidentally, which isn't found in many plants.

FATIGUE: Having plenty folate in your diet can also keep up the energy levels. So if you're tired rather a lot, then this might help give you a boost generally.

INFERTILITY: To return to the subject of zinc, some sources suggest that a deficiency here could be tied to male infertility and as one of the best food sources of zinc is spinach, you know what to do.

TINNITUS: Again, in some instances, tinnitus can also be linked to this kind of deficiency. While this may not be true in all cases, it's certainly worth a try if you have continual or recurring tinnitus.

A WORD OF CAUTION: I can't think of any, although of course if you start experiencing Popeye-like symptoms and socking everyone in sight, do let me know!

INTERESTING FACT: Popeye was invented to encourage people to eat spinach during the Second World War when food was rationed and many things were in short supply.

Sunflower

Sunflower isn't just a pretty flower to look at, the seeds contain many properties, while the oil can be used as a base to which other oils can be added, making them easier to massage into the skin. One of the properties that sunflower seeds contain is that they are largely anti-inflammatory, which is good news for arthritic sufferers. They also contain vitamin E, so a handful in the diet daily can do no harm.

SEEDS

ARTHRITIS: You would have to eat a lot of seeds to get the full benefit of the properties in sunflower. But I do believe that changing your diet, if you have a particular condition, can help. This is one change I'd therefore recommend if you suffer from arthritis. Ask at your health shop.

INFERTILITY: One of the compounds in sunflower seeds is also recommended for men with low sperm counts. If this is you, then you might find that eating a teaspoonful of sunflower seeds each day could improve this condition. Velvet beans, Brazil nuts, chives and peanuts, also contain this compound.

PAIN: Sunflower seeds can help relieve pain. You can try mashing them up and making them into a poultice or eating a handful.

OIL

BURNS: Sunflower oil can help relieve the pain of a burn if applied to the affected area, as well as reducing the chances of the skin blistering.

TENDINITIS: Add some drops of rosemary or sage oil to a tablespoonful of sunflower oil and rub it in to reduce the pain of this condition. (See Tendinitis, page 105.)

A WORD OF CAUTION: So far as I know, sunflower seeds and oil are safe to use for the above conditions. Obviously, if you find they disagree with you, or if you experience any kind of allergic reaction, then discontinue use.

INTERESTING FACT: All parts of the sunflower can be useful for different things. The flowers as a dye and the leaves as fodder.

Tea tree oil

Once again we have the Australian aborigines to thank for

discovering the uses of this helpful oil. It was they who originally discovered its benefits when it came to treating skin infections, cuts and scrapes. In addition to healing the skin, tea tree oil also reduces the likelihood of scarring. But let's not get too carried away! Tea tree oil should not be swallowed, put round the eyes or on sensitive skin because, in some cases, it can irritate. Like everything else, it has to be used according to instructions.

Personally speaking, I don't have a great amount of tea tree oil in my home, not because I dislike or distrust it, rather that I had a very unpleasant and frightening experience with it. My then three-month-old daughter Athena had a nasty bout of cradle cap and, thinking I was doing the best thing, I stupidly poured a few drops of tea tree oil directly onto her scalp. It of course proceeded to run down her forehead into her eyes. The poor wee soul was clearly in agony as she screamed out in pain. I first phoned my GP who told me to get her to Accident and Emergency at once. A few minutes later he called back to say that he had telephoned the poisonous substance unit at one of the big London hospitals (this naturally did nothing to alleviate my fears!) and they too advised that she be admitted to hospital at once! Before making a mad dash to the car, I poured almost an entire jug of water onto my already disturbed baby, thus causing her to become even more disturbed. However, this was the best course of immediate action as the water was to flush out as much of the oil as possible. Thankfully all was well in the end and we got Athena home after she was checked out by a doctor. I shall, however, never forget my experience with tea tree oil, believe in it as I do!

Here are a few good tips where tea tree oil is beneficial, used correctly of course!

DANDRUFF: Tea tree oil contains an antiseptic that not only penetrates the top layer of the scalp but carries deeper than many shampoos. So try mixing a few drops of oil with a herbal shampoo each time you wash your hair. The scalp should stop flaking and heal. Alternatively, you could look at the range of herbal shampoos to see if any contain tea tree.

HEAD LICE: Used regularly tea tree oil can also reduce head lice.

CANDIDA: Tea tree oil is also good for curing candida and other vaginal yeast infections. Either ask in your health shop for suppositories, or mix two or three drops in a tablespoon of yoghurt, then soak a tampon in it. Insert tampons as many times as necessary, until the condition is cleared. However, remember that tampons should be removed and a new one inserted every four hours due to the danger of toxic shock syndrome. And never apply tea tree oil directly onto the vagina or surrounding areas.

CUTS, SCRAPES, BLEMISHES, BITES AND STINGS: These can all be treated with tea tree oil. Many health shops, supermarkets and cosmetic companies now sell tea tree oil sticks which can be used rather like an antiseptic cream, to treat various skin conditions, including acne, and to soothe cuts and bites. No herbal first aid kit should be without one.

PLOOKS (as commonly called in Scotland): Spots or pimples can be made to vanish overnight either by the use of these new tea tree oil sticks found in good chemists or, as I do, by dowsing a cotton bud with oil and then dabbing it onto the offending area.

A WORD OF CAUTION: Never swallow tea tree oil. It is for external use only. And never apply directly onto a three-month-old baby's scalp! Be wary of using tea tree oil on very sensitive skin or on broken skin.

INTERESTING FACTS: In 1770, Captain Cook's sailors brewed a tea from the leaves, thus introducing the name 'tea tree'. It is also said they used it to flavour beer. Actual tea leaves, however, have nothing to do with this particular tree! During the First World War, Australian soldiers caused a huge demand for tea tree oil when it was discovered to be hugely beneficial as a disinfectant. My own tip for this, now that my baby is potty training (and being a tad over the top when it comes to hygiene), is to dilute a few drops of tea tree oil into some previously boiled water, and wash round the potty. Germs, as you know, are renowned for hanging around such areas!

Thyme

Here's another one that we tend to think of mainly as a culinary herb. Yet thyme has a long history and not just as a meat flavouring! In Europe, where it originates, it was used to treat many ailments – laryngitis and whooping cough amongst them. It's just taken us a bit longer to cotton on. Hopefully we will once we see what it can do.

AMENORRHEA: Some herbalists think that thyme can help bring on menstruation, although you would need to combine it with other herbs. Some of these are coriander, fennel, ginger, oregano, parsley, rosemary, catnip and caraway. And what you have to do is put a dash of them in boiling water, allow them to steep for 15 minutes, then strain and drink.

HEADACHE: Thyme tea is reckoned to be a good remedy for treating headaches. Put one teaspoon of dried herb in a cup of boiling water, steep for ten minutes, strain then drink.

BRONCHITIS: Historically, certain of the properties in thyme were thought to ease bronchial spasms and relieve catarrh and recent research has actually borne this out. In one German study, thyme extracts were shown to be as effective as synthetic drugs, which isn't bad, I'd say! Either ask at your health shop for cough medicines containing it or – what could be easier? – make your own tea, as described above and take four times a day.

ASTHMA: If you are an asthma sufferer, then you might do well to follow the instructions above. You might find, too, that regularly adding it to your diet can do no harm either. I'm a great believer in that being the best way to stay fit and healthy, and dried thyme is so easy to come by!

STOMACH PROBLEMS: In 'ye olden days', thyme was used extensively to treat a variety of stomach ailments, including the dreaded hookworm. Its mildly sedative effect means that it is good for relaxing stomach muscles and spasms during an upset. It can also help to relieve wind and generally soothe the digestive tract. If you have an upset try a cup or two of thyme tea. (See above.)

BRUISES AND SPRAINS: Again, for centuries thyme was used to treat both these conditions and thyme baths were used to soothe rheumatic pains. For a bruise, you can try mixing a little thyme oil with some olive oil and applying it to the affected area as often as necessary. For a sprain, it might be appropriate to make a poultice or a compress using dried or fresh thyme. (See our 'How to' section, appendix 4, for how to do this.) Alternatively, you can try making a tea and applying it to the affected area. For aches and pains, put some fresh or dried herb in a small piece of cotton and stitch round. Then let the bath water run through.

WARTS: Here's a real old wife's tale. Just rub some fresh thyme on a wart every day to make it go.

A WORD OF CAUTION: Generally speaking, thyme is a safe herb to use and I have never experienced any problems in using it. As a cough medicine it can be given to children. However, the oil is highly toxic and should never be taken. If you experience any problems in applying the oil or the tea to your skin, then stop using it, as you may be allergic. Otherwise, thyme is safe, easy to find and to use.

INTERESTING FACT: The word is said to derive from the Greek word Thumas, meaning courage.

Uva Ursi

An evergreen shrub, Uva Ursi is lovingly referred to as 'bearberry'. This is, in many ways, an honour to bears, who apparently adore its bright berries. The plant grows in colder climates primarily in Asia. Its principal use is for fighting urinary infections. In fact, up until the early part of the twentieth century, Uva Ursi, due to its quite brilliant ability to fight off and even kill bacteria, was used as a urinary antiseptic.

The green leaves stemming from the plant are formulated into capsules, tinctures and quite often teas (mostly used by the Russians).

WEIGHT LOSS: It is believed, although not proven, that the berries of the Uva Ursi plant act as a beneficial aid to weight loss. However, as this plant is believed to have various adverse affects (see my word of caution), a maximum usage of seven days is recommended.

INFECTIONS (all types): Most parts of the body where infection occurs can benefit by using Uva Ursi. The reason behind this is due to its astringent properties. It largely works as a 'flush out' mechanism.

CYSTITIS: Cystitis and other urinary infections can be treated with Uva Ursi, due to the active ingredients in the plant. Arbutin, one of the greater properties within Uva Ursi, is known to kill bacteria. It is also said that it causes a more fluent flow of water to the kidney, thus literally dissolving the bacteria.

A WORD OF CAUTION: Very few, if any, recorded human tests have to date been carried out on Uva Ursi and its benefits. It is therefore a remedy best taken with complete caution. If symptoms do not begin to improve within a 48-hour period, it is recommended that you cease use of Uva Ursi, as overuse can cause kidney problems. Beware of a strange colour in your urine, in which case – although this is thought to be harmless – it is advisable to reduce the dosage.

Vitamin C and Uva Ursi are *not* the best of friends and mix badly when taken together. Pregnant and nursing woman and anyone with any history of kidney complaints should avoid this remedy. Always follow the manufacturer's instructions to avoid prolonged or over usage of this remedy.

INTERESTING FACTS: Although not generally recommended for the very young, I once prescribed Uva Ursi to a client's ten-year-old daughter who had a problem with bed-wetting. It solved the problem within a matter of days (or rather, nights!).

Valerian

Valerian is a very good herb to take if you can't sleep or are overwrought in general. It's truly unpleasant smell means it's best taken as a tablet, although a tea can be made from the dried root. I just wouldn't recommend it!

ANXIETY AND STRESS: Valerian is very good for relieving anxiety, stress and panic attacks. As it is sleep-inducing, it can be difficult to take during the day, but you could try cutting the dosage, so that way you're still getting a mild relaxing effect and also only use it when you really feel you need to. Stress is often related to the way we live, so have a look at that. Too often we live life to the hilt then expect miracle cures when things go wrong.

INSOMNIA: Let's be honest here, usually at some point or other, we all experience difficulty sleeping. The first thing to do is not to get worked up about it. That's easier said than done, I know, but try to remember sleep patterns do re-establish themselves. A big cause of not sleeping is stress, or worry, or overwork. If you're suffering any of these, then establishing a bedtime routine is as important as swallowing a sleep-inducing drug, then hoping it will do the trick, or falling into bed after a stressful day and expecting to drop off immediately. You won't, because your body's not ready to. Take time to relax, have a herbal bath (see Lavender, page 192), read, wind down, think of nice soothing places to be. This is all just as important and neglected by many sufferers. Taking valerian can certainly help you sleep, as it makes you relax, without giving you that knocked out feeling many medications do.

PRE-MENSTRUAL TENSION: Taking valerian before your period is due could help relieve this condition.

GENERAL ACHES AND PAINS: If you've been overdoing it and are suffering general aches and pains, then a valerian tablet at bedtime could help relax the body overnight, so that you wake in the morning feeling refreshed.

AVAILABILITY: Valerian is available in capsule form from health shops and works best with other sleep-inducing preparations, such as camomile tea. It's safe, easy to take and I certainly don't hesitate to suggest it for people with sleeping problems.

A WORD OF CAUTION: Because of its compounds, valerian may cause drowsiness if taken during the day, so keep it for bedtime. Extremely large doses may cause nausea and dizziness, so don't over do it, no matter how tired you are. And please don't take valerian every night for weeks on end. Valerian isn't addictive but it is important to try to maintain some kind of natural sleep pattern. That said, it is one of my more 'prescribed' supplements. Look out for a daytime version of this supplement as I have been told by a reader that such a product is available.

INTERESTING FACT: Valerian has been used for centuries to help people get a good night's sleep. I've been known on the odd occasion(!) to use it myself.

Vinegar

Vinegar, the plain ordinary sort, is good for quite a few things. Because it's also a preservative, you can also use it to pickle certain of your favourite herbs, then you can add them to your salads whenever you like. All you have to do is steep two teaspoons of dried herb to a litre of vinegar. As a handy remedy to have in the cupboard, however, vinegar is good for the following,

STINGS: If you've nothing else to hand you can safely dab vinegar on a wasp sting to counteract the pain and swelling. It's a very old but tried and tested remedy.

NOSEBLEED: Again, dabbing some vinegar on a wet cotton wool plug and holding it under the nose is reputed to work for nosebleeds, if the person sniffs the vapour.

VAGINITIS: Three cups of apple cider vinegar in a hot bath is supposed to help ease this painful condition, if you soak in it for 20 minutes, letting the water flow into the vagina. Apparently this is because it helps restore normal acidity.

DANDRUFF: Apple juice was traditionally used to treat dandruff, so I wouldn't disagree with this one. Apply warm vinegar to the scalp, then shampoo. Apple cider vinegar is also reputed to be good and is used in exactly the same way.

BODY ODOUR: Not only does bathing in apple cider vinegar help with vaginitis, it also helps with this problem. Although don't expect it to if you have this because your hygiene isn't what it should be! This is for those who tend to sweat a lot. Add a cupful to your bath. Generally, apple cider vinegar and plain vinegar contain antiseptic qualities, so they are good for skin care.

SUNBURN: The same goes for sunburn as for body odour. A cup of apple cider vinegar in your bath should ease that prickly sensation.

ARTHRITIS: This is a really old one, but a teaspoonful of apple cider vinegar in hot water with a spoonful of honey each morning is supposed to help prevent arthritis and I have heard it said that it can also help keep it under control. Some people mix it with molasses instead. Either way so many people swear by it, it's worth a try.

A WORD OF CAUTION: Personally I don't know of anyone who has suffered ill effects from using vinegar. Obviously it's not the kind of thing anyone is going to be silly enough to drink in huge quantities and sprinkling it on food is a good way to take it in any case, especially when it's mixed with herbs. It's also a good cheap remedy to have in the cupboard for certain small emergencies!

INTERESTING FACT: No doubt Jack's head really was made better when he fell down the hill. Traditionally, vinegar and brown paper did more than wrap fish suppers. It was, in fact, quite a plaster cast in its own right a few hundred years ago!

Violet

Whenever I mention using violets to cure certain ailments, I am aware of people looking at me as if I have suddenly sprouted two heads, four legs, six ears, as many arms and taken to dancing about the streets. That's because people tend to think of them as a pretty plant or perfume. At least I hope that's why they are looking at me strangely! Of course violets *are* nice plants, but they have healing powers too. That's why I have a clump or two of them in my garden. Here are some of the things I've found them good for.

HAYFEVER: If you can't stop sneezing and your eyes are beginning to feel like ping-pong balls twanging around in your head, then try boiling a kettle of water, pouring it in a basin with a handful each of marsh mallow flowers and violets, placing a towel over your head and inhaling. I should hope the result would be fairly instant.

HEADACHE: Traditionally, violet tea was used to cure a sore head and even in cases of migraine, violet tea can help with the headache as it also contains a gentle relaxant. So if your sore head is stress induced, then this is one remedy for you. If you can't find a ready bagged tea, then you can add a handful of flowers to a cup of boiling water, strain then drink.

VARICOSE VEINS: Some herbalists even cite violets as being good for this condition and frankly I'd agree. They contain a substance that strengthens the vein walls. If you are a sufferer I'd ask at your health shop for teas containing violet or think about making your own (see above). Violets are an edible flower.

A WORD OF CAUTION: So far as I know violets are safe to take, so long as you don't go mad, trying to eat the whole plant! Seriously, herbal remedies should be used according to instruction and not overdosed on.

INTERESTING FACT: Violets are supposed to carry the image of the face of Jesus.

Vitamins

Vitamins are absolutely essential to our daily wellbeing, whether it's fighting disease or keeping our body parts fit and in good working order. Yet we often get muddled about what does what, where to get it and how much we need. I've tried to simplify this, so you'll know. You'll also know if you have a deficiency! I hope not. But if you do, you'll also know what to do.

VITAMIN A

WHERE IS IT FOUND? Vitamin A is naturally found in dairy products, liver and that old bugbear – cod liver oil! Also, substances that contain beta-carotene can help provide us with vitamin A because the body can convert it (see Beta-carotene, page 133). Carrots are a good source of beta-carotene.

WHAT DOES IT DO? Generally, vitamin A looks after the cells, helps keep down infections and makes sure that bones and bodies grow properly. So making sure we are not deficient keeps our immune systems working properly and helps to ensure that our bodies are producing the protein we need.

COULD YOU BE DEFICIENT? If you are eating insufficient foods containing it, then yes. Remember, diet is a very important part of keeping fit and healthy. If for any reason you do not eat the foods mentioned above, or cannot, then it is important to consider taking supplements. Deficiency symptoms include dry skin, poor night vision and infections.

WHAT CONDITIONS CAN IT HELP? Infections and skin conditions.

A WORD OF CAUTION: The problem with vitamins is getting the balance right. Some people charge around, eating what they like and don't take enough, while others are over zealous and take too much. Too much vitamin A can cause headaches, fatigue and bone problems. Pregnant women shouldn't go above the daily recommended dose.

THE SENSIBLE THING? Try to get enough vitamins from your food in the first place, if not, look at the supplements available and take the recommended dose. That should keep you generally healthy.

VITAMIN B6

WHERE IS IT FOUND? And you thought there was only one vitamin B! Well, there's not, and this one is found in potatoes, bananas, liver, tuna, turkey and lentils.

WHAT DOES IT DO? Vitamin B6 processes the amino acids, the things we all need to make protein. It also makes melatonin and is essential to regulating our moods and mental processes. As with vitamin B12 it keeps one of the amino acids down, one that has been linked to heart disease, stroke and Alzheimer's disease.

COULD YOU BE DEFICIENT? Actual deficiencies are very rare, since the foods this vitamin is found in pretty well cross the board. Alcoholics, patients with kidney failure and women taking oral contraceptives can be deficient, however. The symptoms are mental confusion, skin troubles and generally feeling run down. Although actual deficiencies are rare, many nutritionists don't think we get enough B6 from food. It's not a question of being deficient. It's a question of taking more.

WHAT CONDITIONS DOES IT HELP? Depression, acne, attention deficit disorder, asthma, and pre-menstrual tension.

A WORD OF CAUTION: If you are pregnant or breast-feeding, you shouldn't take more than 100 mg a day in supplement form. Too high levels can also cause damage to the sensory nerves, leading to numbness in the hands and feet and difficulty walking. So, as we don't all want to be wheelchair bound because we're popping our B6s, this is something to consider. If these symptoms develop, stop taking supplements. You'll find the dosage instructions on the packet. Stick to them.

THE SENSIBLE THING: If you're taking the nutritionists' advice and taking supplements because you feel your diet is poor or you want to get more B6, perhaps with the intention of reducing the risk of certain conditions, then please be sensible about what I've just said. There's no point making the second state worse than the first, by developing another condition in order to 'cure' the one you might not even have! This goes for all things generally.

VITAMIN B12
WHERE IS IT FOUND? Dairy foods, eggs, meat, fish and poultry.

WHAT DOES IT DO? Like many other vitamins, vitamin B12 is needed for keeping the cells functioning properly. It also works with folic acid to control levels of a very grand-sounding thing called homocysteine. Put simply, too much of the grand-sounding thing and you're in trouble. Homocysteine is an amino acid and, as such, necessary to the body's well being. Excesses increase the risk of stroke and heart disease. So we need our B12 to keep it in abeyance. It's as simple as that.

COULD YOU BE DEFICIENT? You'd only have to take a brief glance at the above list to know that vegans are very likely to be deficient. The elderly, and sufferers of pernicious anaemia, can also be quite badly deficient, so if you're in these categories, the answer is yes. The symptoms to look out for are fatigue, lack of energy, depression – because it also produces mood-altering substances – and anaemia. Just because you haven't got anaemia doesn't mean you're not suffering a deficiency, incidentally.

WHAT CONDITIONS DOES IT HELP? Depression, pernicious anaemia, fatigue, male infertility.

A WORD OF CAUTION: I can't personally think of any, except to say that if you do have any of the conditions listed above you would have to think in terms of taking vitamin B12 injections rather than supplements. The body's ability to absorb large amounts taken orally is poor.

THE SENSIBLE THING: Most people don't actually need to take supplements because they get enough from their diet. If you're in that category then fine. If not, you can supplement your diet with vitamin tablets. As with all things, be sensible and take them according to the dosage instructions.

VITAMIN C

WHERE IS IT FOUND? Vitamin C is found in many foods. The best sources are broccoli, parsley, citrus fruits, strawberries, currants and Brussels sprouts.

WHAT DOES IT DO? Well, lots would be the answer here! First of all it is an antioxidant which means that it protects us from damage. In particular, it protects our natural cholesterol from becoming damaged and our livers as well, from all the alcohol we pour through them! It also strengthens the blood and muscles, and heals wounds. It can reduce the severity of a cold and some recent research also suggests that it keeps the heart healthy and reduces some of the damage done by diabetes.

COULD YOU BE DEFICIENT? I hope not! But smokers have lower levels and may need to take supplements. Signs of deficiency are fatigue, bleeding gums and easy bruising.

WHAT CONDITIONS CAN IT HELP? Angina, bronchitis, colds, sore throats, glaucoma, infection, male infertility, wound healing.

A WORD OF CAUTION: Very high levels can deplete the body of copper and cause diarrhoea, so don't go mad! If you're taking a supplement, follow the dosage instructions. If you have kidney stones you should avoid supplements. However, I remember being told by my GP that overdosing on vitamin C would cause only a 'straight through' process, meaning it would go in one end and come out the other, doing no damage in the process.

THE SENSIBLE THING: Well, as I've already said, you should try to eat food containing this and other vitamins on a daily basis. The body does not store vitamin C – unfortunately – so even if you're taking a supplement, it won't build up. You can, however, be healthy by making sure you include the above foods in your diet. In terms of preventing disease, even a small daily amount is helping do the trick. I have always found 1 g (1,000 mg) is a safe amount to take and if I feel the onset of a cold coming on, I double the dosage to 2,000 mg. You can buy high-strength vitamin C very easily – in general the highest level I've found is 1,500 mg.

VITAMIN D

WHERE IS IT FOUND? Traces of vitamin D are found in egg yolks and butter as well as cod liver oil. However, most vitamin D is created by being in the sun. But bear in mind the constant warnings we receive these days about spending too long in the sun. It seems only a certain amount of sunlight is good for us in our daily lives. That can be difficult in the UK, which is why some of us feel a bit low at the end of the winter.

WHAT DOES IT DO? Vitamin D keeps calcium in the body and therefore spares the bones having to substitute theirs. It will also transfer calcium from the bones where there is a deficiency – something that doesn't do the bones any favours. Vitamin D is necessary for healthy bones and teeth.

COULD YOU BE DEFICIENT? If you are a strict vegetarian, then you are at more risk. Deficiencies are also more common among the elderly. Dark-skinned people, alcoholics and those with liver or kidney conditions also are more prone to deficiencies. If you have liver or kidney disease then your body can make vitamin D but it cannot get it going. What I said about the sun wasn't a joke. Generally, too, people are more deficient at the end of winter. Deficiencies can cause abnormal bone formation.

WHAT CONDITIONS DOES IT HELP? Generally, by keeping the bones healthy we are lessening our chances of getting bone conditions such as osteoporosis. It can be used to help rickets.

A WORD OF CAUTION: Too much, taken for long periods of time in supplement form, can lead to headaches, weight loss and kidney stones. If your blood level of calcium is already high – and, believe me, you would know about this from your doctor already – you should not take vitamin D supplements, without consulting your doctor first. Remember too, if you're going to get yours from the sun, to use proper sunscreen and be sensible in terms of the time you spend out in the sun. Skin cancer is on the increase in the UK and even putting that risk aside, sunburn is very unpleasant. I know. I've done it. Try to stay out of the sun when the rays are at their most dangerous, which is generally between noon and 2 p.m.

THE SENSIBLE THING: People who spend plenty of time in the sun and eat the right food, don't require supplements. So try to make sure you do both. If you can't and you want to keep your bones healthy, then try a supplement. Nowadays they come with other vitamins, which makes this easy. Remember to follow the dosage instructions.

VITAMIN E

WHERE IS IT FOUND? Vitamin E is found in lots of foods. Nuts, whole grains, egg yolks, vegetable oil, seeds and green leafy vegetables.

WHAT DOES IT DO? This vitamin is also a powerful antioxidant. It helps protect the cells and reduce the risk of heart disease, which is good news for those who feel they are at risk.

COULD YOU BE DEFICIENT? Actual deficiencies are rare. So now you're asking why heart disease exists, if taking vitamin E can reduce the risk and we're all getting enough? The answer is – ah, but are we? Although vitamin E is found in many foods, the levels found in supplements are much higher. If you are worried about the possibility of heart disease and want to keep your body healthy generally, then you should perhaps consider taking them.

WHAT CONDITIONS DOES IT HELP? Vitamin E can help boost the immune system generally, as well as reducing the risk of heart disease. Osteoarthritis, minor injuries, diabetes – oh, and sunburn. So if you've sat in the sun too long trying to get your vitamin D, it's very useful!

A WORD OF CAUTION: Supplements are generally considered to be safe. So far as I am aware I have never heard of anyone suffering side effects from this vitamin.

THE SENSIBLE THING: Keep eating the food mentioned above and it's sure to be good for you. But if you want to get more, then add supplements and take them according to the instructions.

VITAMIN K

WHERE IS IT FOUND? Vitamin K can be acquired from food, particularly leafy green vegetables. But it mainly comes from healthy bacteria in the intestines.

WHAT DOES IT DO? Like many other vitamins, vitamin K helps promote strong bones. It can also help prevent excessive bleeding.

COULD YOU BE DEFICIENT? Since most of this vitamin is produced by our own bodies, in accordance with our needs, this is unlikely.

WHAT CONDITIONS CAN IT HELP? Because it keeps the bones healthy, supplements of vitamin K can help with osteoporosis.

A WORD OF CAUTION: Vitamin K supplements can interfere with other medications, particularly those that thin the blood, such as warfarin and aspirin, if you are taking the latter on a long-term basis. If you are taking vitamin K as part of a multi-vitamin pill, then it is safe, on the whole. But if you are taking it in higher doses, you should consult your doctor first. Please also consult your doctor if you are pregnant or breast-feeding and are thinking of taking vitamin K supplements. In high doses it can cause sweating and flushing. Also, high doses of vitamins E and K don't go too well together. You might find that really high amounts of vitamin E actually increase the risk of bleeding, so that's something else to think about, if you are taking both.

THE SENSIBLE THING: This is one vitamin that might be best taken as a supplement only if you really need to. Otherwise stick to what the body produces, or the dose that comes as part of a multi-vitamin pack.

Walnut

Walnut trees have their uses and it's not just for making furniture. The nuts are delicious and full of things that are good for us. Some studies even suggest that they are so filling they might actually help you lose weight, although nuts don't come in for that kind of praise generally! So all these chocolate-coated ones you've munched your way through might actually be doing quite the opposite of what you expected! Who knows! The leaves and shells are good, too, for treating one or two things. In fact it's the use of these that I am going to look at here.

SCABIES: Walnut shells can help treat this irritating skin condition caused by mite infestation. Boil the cracked shell pieces in a cup of water until half the water is evaporated. Cool, drain, and then apply the liquid to the skin. The chemicals contained in the shell soon get rid of the mites.

SKIN PROBLEMS: Walnut leaves are useful for treating minor skin infections. You can either add a handful of crushed leaves to your bath water, or steep the leaves in boiling water, cool, drain, then apply the liquid to the skin.

A WORD OF CAUTION: If you suffer from a nut allergy, please stay clear of walnuts and their shells. Consult your doctor about using any of the treatments mentioned here. Otherwise, walnuts are safe to take and you should suffer no ill effects from using their leaves.

INTERESTING FACTS: The name walnut means 'foreign nut'. The tree is thought to have been introduced to Britain by the Romans but was not cultivated for centuries. A tree will not produce nuts until it is over 20 years old.

Wintergreen

This little herb is not readily available at herbalists, although it can generally be ordered. I just love its name. Being 'awfully poetic', it just gives you a little hope, even to hear it! Wintergreen is a sort of herbal aspirin and, as such, is good for the things that aspirin is good for, like headache and flu, colds, aches and general pains. I also recommend it for:

AMENORRHEA: There are many herbs that can help bring on menstrual flow. Wintergreen is one. You could try steeping it in boiling water for 15 minutes, then drinking the cooled liquid. Other commonly available herbs which you could try adding a dash of – and I do stress the word 'dash' – are coriander, fennel, ginger, oregano, parsley, thyme, rosemary, tansy, tarragon, lemon balm, lavender and that Victorian lady's aid, pennyroyal. Phew!

BACKACHE: Oil of wintergreen makes a good external massage oil if you suffer from backache. Wintergreen itself has a rather pleasant taste, so if you're using the oil just be sure that you keep it away from children, and don't take it yourself. The herb is safe and so are tablets and capsules, but oils are for external use only.

EARACHE: A tea made by pouring boiling water over a handful of dried herb can help an earache. Or you can have it handy in tablet form. Just remember what I've said about aspirin. And don't give aspirin-like substances to children, as there's a chance they could develop a rather nasty disease later on that damages the liver and kidneys.

HANGOVER: While aspirin itself can irritate the stomach making it *not* the ideal cure for a hangover, the substances found in wintergreen are far gentler, so it's worth a shot. That's if you've got some handy in the medicine cupboard. Obviously, if you have a hangover you're in no fit state to go looking!

SORE THROAT: Wintergreen has such a pleasant taste I'd recommend you making a tea and gargling with it if you have a sore throat. Just put a teaspoon of dried herb in boiling water, allow it to sit for ten minutes, strain and gargle. The compounds in it should soon go to work and you can repeat every three hours till your throat feels better.

A WORD OF CAUTION: If you're allergic to aspirin or have been told to stay off it, don't take wintergreen. The compounds are the same.

INTERESTING FACT: Wintergreen was used externally for hundreds of years to treat gout.

Witch hazel

Witch hazel is undergoing something of a revival at the moment, I would say, judging by the amount of people who are turning to it for help with skin conditions and to improve the look of their skin generally. It's another of these ones our mothers knew about and their mothers before them. In fact, witch hazel has been used for hundreds of years for many things. It's very easily obtainable from chemists and health shops. I certainly always keep a bottle handy.

BRUISES: Soothe really bad bruises, the ones that are painful to the touch and seem to keep bleeding under the skin, by carefully dabbing some witch hazel on two or three times a day. It certainly heals them quicker. That's because it tones up the blood vessels and gets the blood supply going to the damaged areas.

SKIN PROBLEMS: The same goes for minor skin problems, such as rashes, small irritations, and dermatitis. All you have to do is apply regularly with cotton wool. Sometimes I suggest adding it to acne preparations. A little in a cup of camomile tea – not for drinking by the way – can help soothe the skin, take out the redness, and help the spots heal quicker. It might not chase it away completely, but it certainly seems to bring it under control.

SUNBURN: Aloe Vera is still one of the best things for sunburn. But I used witch hazel on a recent holiday where the Aloe Vera bottle had got crushed – oh, these baggage handlers – and I was out. It wasn't as effective, but it did help. So if you've nothing else, pour a little on a towel and press it on for a while.

VARICOSE VEINS: Witch hazel applied externally can help with varicose veins. That's because it strengthens the blood vessels. So you could try making a compress and pressing it on.

STINGS AND BITES: Apply witch hazel to stings and bites. You could even keep some frozen in the freezer – that's most effective. Just remember if you do make 'ice-cubes' with witch hazel to label them. It really wouldn't do for them to wind up in someone's drink by mistake.

A WORD OF CAUTION: Witch hazel is meant for external use only. Never take it unless you're buying a preparation that says so. I'm saying that because in some instances you can take the tincture or make a tea with the dried leaves. That's not what I'm recommending here, however. So stick to the instructions.

INTERESTING FACT: The name is derived from the use of the twigs of the tree as divining rods.

Yoga

WHAT IS IT? Yoga has been practised for thousands of years and, like many other therapies, it is based on the belief that for the body to be healthy, the mind must play a part. In fact in yoga, the body and mind must be seamlessly connected, as one, so to speak. Harmony, balance and peace are the ultimate aims of this therapy, therefore, rather than a cure for a particular condition. Because it can do certain things it can benefit various ailments, however. The mind has many powers. Ones we've never fully tapped into and many we never use. I sometimes feel that ancient civilisations understood this better and that, as well as being good exercise, yoga is a demonstration of this.

HOW DOES IT WORK? There are different kinds of yoga, which I feel is another benefit. So if you're worried about wrapping your ankles round your neck, you can choose one to suit yourself, so to speak! However, the most widely practised is called Hatha Yoga. It concentrates on breathing, posture and meditation. The breathing helps to focus the mind and is important for relaxation and meditation. While the postures include different things, like standing, balancing and yes, for the more advanced, backward bends. More advanced at the technique, that is, not in age. What you'll find is that you won't be asked to do something you can't. Yoga isn't there to worry you. Quite the opposite. It works by helping you to become more flexible, more focused and calmer.

WHAT DOES IT HELP IN PARTICULAR? Primarily, yoga helps to reduce stress and it promotes the release of the body's natural painkillers. So while it may not 'cure' a condition, as such, it can improve your state of health generally, thus helping the condition to be cured. Yoga is good for insomniacs, and people with digestive problems. It decreases blood pressure, improves the respiratory rate and makes the heart fitter. Some studies have also shown that it's good for people with flexibility problems. It is also recommended for people with depression, migraine, diabetes, cancer, arthritis and asthma. Not bad at all, I would say!

HOW LONG SHOULD A COURSE OF TREATMENT LAST? A class generally lasts 60–90 minutes and beginners should take two a week. How long you continue and how far you go is up to you. Classes usually begin with a period of quiet. The gentle warm up exercises follow. Then the teacher will take you into a series of postures, which you hold for a few seconds. As you get better at it, you learn harder postures and hold them for longer. At the classes you will learn the breathing as you go along. A class usually ends with students lying comfortably on the floor, relaxing.

HOW DO I GO ABOUT GETTING THIS TREATMENT? Well, the beauty of Hatha Yoga is that you can teach yourself from books. To get the full benefit you should really enrol in a class and if you look around I think you'll see that these are often run locally in church halls, community centres and fitness centres.

A WORD OF CAUTION: When you're looking for a class, check out the kind of experience the teacher has and if you're at all unhappy, move on. The best teachers are those with years of experience although that is not to say a new teacher isn't any good. Obviously all teachers differ. Some concentrate more on certain aspects than others. So that gives more scope for you to find someone who suits if, say, you're not in very good shape and you want to concentrate more on the breathing and relaxation to start with. Yoga should be a pleasant experience, so again if you feel you're being rushed through at break-neck speed and coming home with twisted muscles, move on. If you're pregnant, and it's very good to do yoga if you are, make sure the exercises are modified for you and avoid postures that put pressure on the uterus. If you're new to a class, tell your teacher if you have a particular condition. It doesn't do, and I think common sense would tell you that, to be doing upside down postures and headstands if you have a hernia or high blood pressure. Or to be bending over if you have a slipped disc! Nor would that look very good for the teacher if something happened because you hadn't said.

INTERESTING FACT: There is evidence that yoga was practised 5,000 years ago. The first written description of this ancient philosophy dates from the second century BC.

Zinc

Zinc is an essential trace mineral, present in drinking water and certain foods, yet it is amazing how many people fail to get enough of it through their diet. Parsley, spinach, Brussels sprouts, cucumbers, prunes and asparagus are all good natural sources of zinc. Spinach has the most. It is possible to add some of these together to make a soup – see our recipe section at the end of the book (page 261). We hope you'll give it a try, especially when you see some of the benefits!

Severe deficiency is of course rare in the UK, but it's amazing how a host of ills can come about from even a mild one – flu, colds, skin ailments, low blood sugar, low sperm counts, to name a few. So if you're generally run down or suffering continually from any of these things, maybe you aren't getting enough of this mineral. Zinc is believed to boost the immune system. It may even slow the loss of hair, so let's read on and find out the things it can help with.

COLDS AND FLU: When taken right away at the first sign of a runny nose, zinc lozenges can minimise the severity of cold and flu symptoms. In fact, some studies suggest that they cut the length of the infection by a half. Avoid lozenges with citric acid, sorbitol or mannitol. These react with saliva to make zinc ineffective. Suck one lozenge every two hours.

TINNITUS: In some instances a zinc deficiency is thought to be to blame for this troublesome ailment. Eat more vegetables containing zinc, or try a supplement.

GENERAL HEALING: Zinc lozenges not only stave off a sore throat but also make sores heal quicker. Burns, eczema and haemorrhoids all heal quicker if you boost the immune system by taking zinc. So it's an idea to add them to your medicine cabinet and suck them every two hours if you have a sore that isn't healing as well as you would like.

OSTEOPOROSIS. Because it is so good at keeping the bones healthy zinc can help protect against this disease. Many supplement combinations contain zinc with calcium, magnesium and vitamin D – all vital to good bone health – and can be bought in any health store.

ULCERS: Interestingly, people with inflammatory bowel disease are often found to be suffering a zinc deficiency, so zinc may be of use for treating ulcers and other digestive tract problems.

ACNE: Zinc's ability to foster skin healing means that it can be used for acne but it may react with antibiotics. It may also take three to four weeks before you see any result, so don't get your hopes up right away.

FERTILITY: With regard to fertility, or rather the lack of it, zinc promotes proper cell division, the process critical to the earliest stages of conception. Again, studies of male infertility suggest a zinc deficiency can lead to a low sperm count, so get on the soup, the vegetables, or the supplements. You never know – the results may be amazing!

PROSTATE PROBLEMS: Zinc has been shown to reduce the size of the prostate. It ranks among the key nutrients for the health of the prostate gland and is particularly useful for all prostate conditions categorised as mild to moderate. So if you have a weak urine flow or difficulty urinating, you should think about taking supplements. Hopefully it will improve things for you.

EYE PROBLEMS: Problems such as conjunctivitis may also lessen if you take zinc. Since one of zinc's effects is to boost vitamin A, this helps keep eyes generally healthy, in particular the retina. Studies have shown that it can slow vision loss in people with macular degeneration, a common cause of blindness in individuals aged over 50.

WORD OF CAUTION: Zinc, on the whole, is a fairly safe supplement and, as you can see, can be hugely beneficial. However, by taking too much you run the risk of nausea and can also diminish the immune system. Avoid drinking coffee around the time of taking zinc as this can reduce its effectiveness.

INTERESTING FACT: In a study of 118 healthy but elderly residents of an Italian nursing home, researchers found that those given a supplement of 25 mg of zinc every day for three months, were soon leaving their companions behind in the health stakes!

A Few Healthy Recipes

Carrot and coriander soup

INGREDIENTS

1 onion
1 teaspoon dried coriander, or pick fresh if you have it
1 glass of orange juice
Several large carrots, or a good quantity of frozen ones
600 ml chicken or vegetable stock
Salt and black pepper to taste
1 tablespoon of olive oil

1) Chop up the onion and cook in the oil until it is translucent.
2) Pour on the warmed stock. Add the carrots, coriander, and salt and pepper to taste.
3) Bring to the boil and add the orange juice.
4) Cover and simmer for 20 minutes.

Heart soup

INGREDIENTS

50 g unsalted butter
2 large parsnips, diced
2 large onions diced
450 g cooking apples
1 clove garlic
1 large carrot, diced

2 teaspoons medium curry powder
2 teaspoons parsley
1.5 litres chicken/vegetable stock
Salt to flavour

1) Melt the butter in a large pan and sauté the onions and garlic over a low heat until the onions are translucent.
2) Stir in the parsnip, apples and carrot, and sauté for 3 minutes, stirring occasionally.
3) Stir in the parsley and curry powder and sauté for another minute.
4) Pour on the stock. Add salt to flavour and bring to the boil. Cover the pan and simmer for 20 minutes.
5) Puree the soup in a liquidiser or food processor and serve.

Onion soup

INGREDIENTS
3 large onions
1 clove garlic
4 tablespoons olive oil
1 teaspoon dried thyme and sage
1 dried bay leaf
1 litre chicken or vegetable stock
1 tablepoon lemon juice
Salt and black pepper

1) Peel and chop the onions and garlic.
2) Put the olive oil in a large saucepan and cook the onions and garlic until they are translucent.
3) Stir in the herbs.
4) Add the warmed stock, lemon juice, and salt and pepper.
5) Cover and simmer for an hour.

Syrian lentil soup

One way to eat spinach!

INGREDIENTS
200 g lentils
1 litre chicken or vegetable stock
1 large onion
200 g frozen spinach
25 g low fat spread
1 teaspoon lemon juice
Salt

1) Slice the onions and fry gently in melted spread until they are translucent.
2) Remove from the heat and add the lentils, salt and stock.
3) Bring to the boil and simmer for an hour.
4) Add the spinach and simmer for 15 minutes
5) Add the lemon juice before serving.

Zinc soup

It's much better than it sounds!

INGREDIENTS
2 large leeks, chopped
2 large courgettes, chopped
2 large potatoes, peeled and chopped
1 cabbage, chopped
1 teaspoon of parsley
50 g asparagus, chopped
1 tub of cheese spread
2 vegetable stock cubes
Salt to flavour

1) Put the vegetables, parsley and stock cubes in salted water and bring to the boil.

2) When soup is boiling, add the cheese spread, making sure you stir carefully until it has melted.
3) Cover the pan and simmer for 20 minutes.
4) Puree the soup in a liquidiser or food processor and serve.

Carrots in ginger

Variety is the spice of life! The secret's not to put too much water in!

INGREDIENTS
Carrots, 300 g frozen or fresh
1 vegetable stock cube
1 teaspoon of ginger
25 g butter or vegetable spread
Salt to flavour

1) Place the carrots in a saucepan, just covering them with water. Add salt as usual and bring to the boil.
2) When the water is boiling, add the ginger, the butter and the stock cube. Stir and boil for six minutes or until the carrots are soft, watching the pot does not boil dry.

Baked potatoes

INGREDIENTS
4 baked potatoes

FILLING
1 onion, peeled and chopped
4 rashers bacon
175 g mushrooms
1 green pepper, seeded and diced
225 g Cheddar cheese
1 tablespoon wholegrain mustard
2 tablespoons low fat yoghurt
Black pepper

1) Preheat the oven to 220 ºC. Wash the potatoes, then prick them with a fork. Bake for one hour.
2) While potatoes are baking, melt the butter in a large pan and add the onion, bacon and green pepper.
3) Cook for 3 minutes, then add the mushrooms and cook for a further 4 minutes.
4) Remove from the heat. Cut the potatoes in half. Scoop out the insides into a large bowl and mash.
5) Add the vegetable mixture, half the cheese, mustard, black pepper and yoghurt. Mix.
6) Spoon the mixture into potato skins. Sprinkle on the remaining cheese.
7) Return to the oven and bake for 15 minutes. Serve.

Potato cakes

INGREDIENTS
4–6 medium potatoes
26 g low fat spread
Salt and pepper to taste
3 tablespoons milk
50 g flour
2 egg yolks
A little olive oil
Watercress or sliced tomatoes

1) Peel the potatoes and boil in salted water for 20 minutes.
2) Mash up with low fat spread, pinch of pepper and milk.
3) Add the flour and the yolks of the eggs. Mix together well.
4) Heat the olive oil in a frying pan. Put spoonfuls of the mixture in the pan and turn till they are brown on both sides.
5) Serve hot with watercress or tomatoes.

Cheesy vegetables

INGREDIENTS
3 carrots, peeled and sliced
1 cauliflower divided into florets

225 g broccoli
75 g frozen peas

SAUCE
40 g butter
40 g plain flour
450 ml milk
100 g half fat Double Gloucester cheese, grated
2 teaspoons mustard
Salt and black pepper to taste

1) Cook the carrots in boiling water. Add the cauliflower, broccoli and peas. Cook till tender. Drain.
2) Put the vegetables in a large flameproof dish.
3) Melt butter in a pan, add the flour and stir for 1 minute. Remove from the heat and stir in the milk.
4) Return to heat and stir. When thickened add the cheese, mustard, salt and pepper.
5) Pour the sauce over the vegetables and stir. Grill under a medium heat for 5 minutes. Serve.

German cabbage

INGREDIENTS
1 cabbage
1 onion
1 cooking apple
225 g tin of chopped tomatoes
1 litre vegetable stock
Salt and pepper

1) Peel and core the apple and cut up into small pieces. Shred the cabbage. Chop the onion and mix with the apple.
2) Mix the cabbage, onion, apple and tomatoes with the stock and boil it all together for 30 minutes. Season with salt and pepper.

Salad Niçoise

INGREDIENTS
200 g tin of tuna
225 g tin of tomatoes
50 g black olives
2 small onions
Parsley
1 lettuce
4 small cooked potatoes
50 g tin of anchovy fillets
Small cucumber
Vinaigrette dressing
2 hard-boiled eggs

1) Prepare the vegetables by cutting the potatoes into slices, slicing the cucumber, chopping the onions and cutting the tomatoes into eights.
2) Arrange some of the lettuce in a salad bowl. Then arrange the tomatoes and cucumbers in a circle over the lettuce.
3) Sprinkle vinaigrette dressing over this.
4) Place more lettuce on top. Then add a circle of hard-boiled eggs and potatoes.
5) Place more lettuce on top.
6) Drain the oil out of the tuna and add the tuna on top of the salad.
4) Drain the oil from the anchovies and place one or two on top, with the black olives and a sprinkling of onions and parsley.
5) Add more vinaigrette dressing.

Stuffed tomatoes

INGREDIENTS
6 large tomatoes
2 hard-boiled eggs
100 g tinned tuna
Parsley
2 tablespoons mayonnaise
Lettuce leaves

1) Cut a slice off each tomato. Dig out the seeds and liquid with a teaspoon and knife.
2) Chop up the hard-boiled eggs. Shred the tuna and chop the parsley.
3) Mix the egg and tuna together. Add the parsley. Stir in the mayonnaise.
4) Fill the tomatoes with this mixture. Add a dot of mayonnaise and a sprig of parsley.
5) Serve on lettuce leaves.

Nettle beer

This is a traditional gypsy recipe, good for keeping the body fit and healthy so long, of course, as it is only taken in small amounts and not over-consumed!

INGREDIENTS
900 g young nettles
2 lemons
4.5 litres water
450 g brown sugar
25 g cream of tartar
Brewers' yeast, prepared in advance
Plastic bucket and lid

1) Juice the lemons.
2) Put the tops of the nettles in a big saucepan with the lemon rinds. Add the water and bring to the boil. Allow to boil for 20 minutes.
3) Place the sugar and cream of tartar in the bucket then strain the hot liquid onto it. Stir. When it has cooled slightly add the lemon juice and yeast.
4) Cover with the lid and leave to stand in a warm room for three days. Then move to a cooler place and leave for two more days.
5) Syphon into glass bottles. Plastic is no use unless you want exploding nettle beer. If the beer seems to be 'too active' then just loosen the tops slightly for a few days, then tighten. Keep in a cool place for another week before drinking.

Rose petal jelly

Ideal for constipated children!

INGREDIENTS
100 g white rose petals
1 tablespoon lemon juice
2 tablespoons orange juice
2 tablespoons clear honey
450 g white cane sugar
150 ml water

1) Place all the ingredients, except for the petals, in a stainless steel pan and leave to stand until the sugar dissolves.
2) Add the rose petals and heat gently, stirring constantly.
3) Stop when the petals seem to dissolve.
4) Allow to cool.
5) Pour into a jar and seal when cold. Give a teaspoonful when necessary.

Strawberry ice-cream

Deliciously sinful we must admit, but what a way to take your fruit!

INGREDIENTS
Two bowlfuls wild strawberries, washed
Juice of half a lemon
125 g castor sugar
284 ml carton double cream

1) Put the berries and the sugar in a stainless steel pan and heat over a moderate heat, stirring, until the sugar has dissolved and the berries are scenting the air.
2) Pull yourself away from the smell and pour the mixture into a liquidiser.
3) When liquidised, add lemon juice, cover and chill in the fridge for 2 hours.

4) When firmish, whisk in cream and freeze for 6 hours.
5) Eat!

Mint sorbet

INGREDIENTS
400 g caster sugar
345 ml water
3 stalks of fresh mint, chopped
250 ml water
200 ml dry white wine
2 tablespoons lemon juice

1) Put the sugar and 345 ml water in a pan and heat until the sugar dissolves.
2) Bring to the boil and simmer for 5 minutes, then add the mint and 250 ml water.
3) Remove from the heat, add the wine and leave to cool.
4) Chill overnight in the fridge.
5) Add the lemon juice.
6) Freeze for two hours, then remove from the freezer and whisk, using a fork or hand whisk, until smooth.
7) Return to the freezer for 4 hours.

Cranberry fudge

Not for the faint hearted! The secret is in the stirring!

INGREDIENTS
900 g granulated sugar
50 g unsalted butter
1 tablespoon golden syrup
175 ml milk
200 g can full cream condensed milk
100 g fresh cranberries

1) Place the sugar, butter, milk and golden syrup in a saucepan and bring slowly to the boil, stirring all the time.

2) Pour in the condensed milk and boil for 20 minutes, or until the mixture seems to start darkening slightly, stirring constantly. You can test if it's ready by dropping a spoonful in a cup of cold water. If it hardens then remove from the heat.
3) Stir in the cranberries and pour into a greased Swiss roll tin or flan dish. Mark the squares out.
4) When the fudge is cold, break into pieces and store. (That's if you don't eat it first!)

Cranberry tart

Not for the diet conscious!

INGREDIENTS
750 g fresh cranberries
2 x 20 cm shortcrust baked pie shells
150 ml water
3 sachets gelatine crystals
350 g redcurrant jelly
2 teaspoons brandy
225 g granulated sugar

1) Pour the water into a bowl, sprinkle on the gelatine and stand the container in a pan of hot water. Stir until the crystals have dissolved.
2) Put the cranberries, sugar and jelly in a pan and heat gently for 10 minutes, until the fruit is tenderly bubbling but not bursting open. Remove and leave to cool slightly.
3) Stir in the gelatine mixture and the brandy.
4) Cover the fruit with a piece of wet, non-stick baking paper. Allow to cool.
5) Stir the filling and pour into the pie shells. Chill in fridge before serving.

Fruit platter

INGREDIENTS
2 large oranges, peeled
1 peach, stoned and diced
Half a watermelon, made into balls
Half a cantaloupe melon, peeled and cut into wedges
Half a honeydew melon, peeled and cut into wedges
225 g seedless grapes
Sprig of mint

FOR THE DIP
100 g low fat soft cheese
300 ml Greek yoghurt
1 teaspoon finely grated lime rind
2 tablespoons reduced-sugar marmalade
2 teaspoons crystallised ginger
1 teaspoon grated lemon rind

1) Divide the oranges into segments. Arrange on a large flat dish. Do the same with the other fruit and garnish with the mint.
2) Cover with cling film and chill.
3) For the dip. Put the cheese in a mixing bowl. Beat with a mixer. Beat in the yoghurt, lime rind and marmalade.
4) Chop the ginger and stir into the mixture.
5) Spoon into a bowl. Cover with cling film. Garnish with the lemon rind. Chill for one hour.
6) Serve with fruit.

Muesli

Make your own!

INGREDIENTS
4 tablespoons porridge oats
5 tablespoons single cream
1 apple
Grated nuts

1 tablespoon raisins or sultanas, chopped

1) Put everything, except the apple, in a bowl and mix them together to make a liquidy porridge.
2) Cut the apple into quarters without peeling it. Core the quarters. Grate the apple straight onto the muesli.

Old Wives' Tales That Can Work

WRINKLES: Aloe Vera plants can give you a natural facelift, just cut a leaf and rub the cut end into wrinkle areas. Keep the leaf in the fridge till all the moisture is used. After a few weeks you will be amazed at the difference and feel to your skin. Aloe juice is also an excellent soothing remedy for minor burns.

COLD AND SHIVERY, FLU OR COLDS: Soak your feet in a basin of hot water and mustard. It warms the feet and the blood and helps to warm the soul. Physiologically, or whatever, it makes you feel better.

Colds, flus and viruses can be avoided or kept to a minimum by taking vitamin C and zinc regularly when you are exposed to infection or are in the company of a sufferer. As with all vitamins, only take these when needed, have a break and allow the body to go it alone and build up its own immunity. During the winter period take these continually and even double the dose if you are exposed to infection. They don't have any side effects.

TIREDNESS AND STRESS: Run a warm/hot bath and add a few drops of lavender oil, soak for 10 to 15 minutes and then go to bed relaxed and able to sleep. Add a few drops of lavender to the pillow for further relaxation.

INSOMNIA: No need for sleeping pills – try camomile tea with a teaspoonful of honey. Ovaltine, cocoa or Horlicks with a small measure of sherry, port, brandy or whisky added makes a comforting nightcap.

WASP AND BEE STINGS: These respond well to applications of vinegar and internally to rid the body of venom, a drink of warm/hot water with a teaspoonful of cider vinegar and honey added. This should be taken first thing in the morning and last thing in the evening until no signs or swellings are left. Applications of ice can initially reduce swelling from stings

ALLERGIES: These respond well to vitamin B6, which helps the body increase its own supply of antihistamine, unlike antihistamine pills, which stop the body's production of antihistamine. Take one 3–4 times a day, gradually decreasing till symptoms disappear – no falling asleep either.

WATER RETENTION: Nature's natural diuretics, such as cinnamon, turnip, celery, onion, leek and dandelion added to food can help the body against water retention. Vitamin B6 tablets also give good results and have no side effects.

TUMMY UPSET OR GASTRIC FLU/VIRUS: Eat only plain boiled rice and fresh vegetables, except tomatoes, for a speedy recovery. Avoid products that contain a lot of wheat that will stress the 'not so good' tummy and intestines.

HEADACHES THAT DON'T RESPOND TOO QUICKLY TO PAINKILLERS: Put some ice in a plastic bag. Cover with a tea towel and place at the base of the skull.

PAINKILLERS NOT WORKING EFFECTIVELY: Don't increase the dosage – try a vitamin B6 tablet with your pain killer, it can double the effect without doubling the dosage of the painkillers.

BURNS TO FINGERS: Place your finger on your ear lobe and watch how the initial fierce pain of burnt fingers subsides. Works wonders.

BRUISED FINGERS: Fingers caught in a car door, or jammed in any way, can cause a throbbing pain – we've all experienced it, I'm sure. Reduce the pain by putting the finger/s in your mouth, the heat of your breath soothes the throbbing pain.

HAIR: A tablespoon of brown vinegar in the rinsing water for dark hair gives a squeaky clean shine.

PERIOD AND STOMACH PAINS: Breathing deeply and panting (as if giving birth) can be used to treat and eliminate period pains and stomach pains. You concentrate on your deep breathing and when the pain peaks you start shallow panting, going back to the deep breathing as the pain subsides. This is also very effective for cramp in any part of the body. The results steadily improve with practice.

NAUSEA: Ginger, in any form, can ease nausea and sickness. A glass of ginger ale can work wonders for travel sickness.

SKIN RASHES: Adding a handful of Epsom Salts to the bath water can soothe irritated skin or rashes. Never have the water too hot if the skin is irritated in any way.

ULCERS AND MOUTH/GUM INFECTIONS: These respond quickly to using a mouthwash of one teaspoonful of salt and one teaspoonful of bicarbonate of soda in half a cup of water as hot as can be tolerated. Hold in the mouth for as long as possible. This should give approximately 4–5 mouthfuls. This is a useful mouthwash after tooth extraction or injury and will encourage natural healing without infection.

BOOST THE IMMUNE SYSTEM: Adding garlic to cooking can help boost the immune system against minors ailments and the regular eating of garlic can prevent bites by midges and other biting insects.

LOW CHOLESTEROL: Porridge is one of the best foods you can eat, as it keeps cholesterol low and gives energy without being fattening. Many people swear by porridge in the winter as the best warmer of all. Adding a tablespoonful of honey acts as an aid to digestion as well as adding flavour.

FRESH BREATH: The quickest natural way of eliminating garlic and onion breath odours is to chew a few sprigs of fresh parsley.

FOR CRAMP AND/OR A GOOD NIGHT'S SLEEP: At bedtime, take three tablespoonfuls of runny honey in a glass of buttermilk, flavoured with the juice of one lemon.

TO LESSEN THE CHANCE OF ARTHRITIS: Crush half an aspirin and mix this with a spoonful of cider vinegar, a spoonful of honey and a spoonful of hot water and take every day.

TO SOOTHE PAINFUL JOINTS: Put a sprinkling of any three of the following into a base oil such as olive oil and massage into the affected area – garlic, juniper, lavender, sage, rosemary, thyme.

TO MAKE LINIMENT FOR ARTHRITIS: Take two drops of essential oil of cloves, three drops of oil of wintergreen, five drops of oil of camphor and three drops of essential oil of eucalyptus. Mix together and apply.

CATARRH: Drink cabbage juice, coupled with crisp, raw cabbage.

WATER RETENTION: Eat lots of raw celery.

HEADACHE: Smother a medium-sized cooked potato in a sauce made from simmered tinned tomatoes, lots of basil and a dash of vinegar. Then eat. Or find a sweet-smelling leaf. Rub it on your fingers and inhale deeply.

HOW TO MAKE A HEADACHE PILLOW: Mix 50 g lavender, 50 g rose petals 50 g marjoram 50 g rose leaves and 12 g cloves together. Sew into a cotton square and place underneath your pillow.

TO GET RID OF NAUSEA AND A HEADACHE: Mix one level teaspoon each of camomile, mint and catnip tea in a pint of boiled cooled water.

TO DEAL WITH A MIGRAINE: Chew candied Angelica regularly.

The Ideal Home Medical Kit

Well, so you've looked at all this and with the best will in the world you still don't know where to start, or you do but you can't remember all of it. Well that's what these pages are for – to make up your own home medical kit. All I'm doing here is giving you pointers towards the most common ailments. It's up to you what you choose to use.

IDEALLY YOU SHOULD HAVE:
Something antiseptic for cuts, scrapes and bruises.
Some lozenges and herbal remedies for colds and flu.
A selection of teas to help you to relax and sleep.
Various remedies for stomach upset (i.e. diarrhoea, constipation, nausea, indigestion). These could include some teas.
Something for headache, earache, and general aches and pains.
Any supplements/vitamins you feel you may need.
Anything for a particular condition you or members of your family have, or are worried about getting.

Of course this is in addition to foods and herbs you might like to keep handy or add to your diet. The following pages are for that.

How To . . .

Okay we've talked a lot about them – poultices, infusions and tinctures. But maybe you'd like to get right into this by learning how to do these things for yourself. So here's a quick and easy guide on how to go about it.

Poultices

1. Making sure you have enough to cover the affected area, chop up the fresh herb unless it is already in small pieces.
2. Place the herbs in a saucepan.
3. Cover them with a little water and simmer for a few minutes.
4. Squeeze out the moisture and place the simmered herbs on the affected area.
5. Cover with a bandage or strip of cotton and keep in place for 3–4 hours, replacing with a fresh poultice when necessary.

Tinctures

Use either 200 g dried herb or 40 g fresh to 1 litre alcohol/water mix. For alcohol, use either brandy or vodka, adding 1 cup of water to 2 cups alcohol. The resulting mixture will keep for up to two years, so although this might seem expensive, it's not. Obviously a tincture contains a very concentrated dose of the herb, not to mention the fact it's alcohol preserved. So do not give to children and only use where recommended and for short periods of time.

1. Put the herb in a large jar.
2. Pour on the alcohol/water mix.
3. Seal up the jar and place in a cool place for two weeks, making sure you shake the jar every now and then.
4. Pour the mixture through a jelly bag into a clean jug.
5. Squeeze out the tincture from the bag.
6. Pour the strained tincture into bottles. Seal and keep in a cool dry place.

Infusions/teas

1. Place the herb in a cup.
2. Pour in boiling water.
3. Leave to infuse for ten minutes.
4. Strain into another cup.
5. Anything left over can be stored in the fridge for up to two days.

Decoctions

This is for the roots and flowers of a plant, which are far harder to boil into an infusion.

1. Place the herb in a saucepan.
2. Pour on cold water.
3. Bring to the boil and simmer until the liquid is reduced by a third.
4. Strain into a jug and store in a fridge for up to three days.

Stockist List

There are good stockists all over the country, but here are the details of three which I use regularly:

HERBS SCOTLAND
30 Middleton Close
Bridge of Don
Aberdeen
AB22 8HU
Tel: 01224 822374
Fax: n/a
E-mail:
info@herbsscotland.co.uk
Website:
www.herbsscotland.co.uk

NATURE'S WAY
27 High Street East
Ansthruther
Fife
KY10 3DQ
Tel: 01333 311077
Fax: n/a
E-mail:
sj.naturesway@virginnet.co.uk
Website: n/a

PARK ROAD PHARMACY
405 Great Western Road
Glasgow
G4 9HY
Tel: 0141 339 5979
Fax: 0141 337 6900
E-mail:
info@parkroadpharmacy.co.uk
Website:
www.chemist.uk.com

Glossary of Good Health

A

ABSCESSES
Aloe Vera – Echinacea – Root garlic – Goldenseal – Marsh mallow – Myrrh

ACNE
Burdock – Echinacea – Evening primrose oil – Garlic – Red clover – Vitamin B complex

ADENOIDS
Cleavers – Echinacea – Garlic – Goldenseal – Marigold

ALTITUDE SICKNESS
Charcoal tablets – Ginger capsules – Lavender inhalant – Peppermint – Vitamin B2

ANAEMIA
Camomile – Dandelion – Fenugreek – Kelp – Nettle juice – Vitamin C

ANXIETY
Bach's Rescue Remedy – Californian poppy – Camomile – Hyssop – St John's Wort – Valerian

APPETITE LOSS
Blessed thistle – Californian poppy root – Camomile – Goldenseal – Tansy – Vitamin B complex

ARTHRITIS
Bittersweet – Burdock – Celery – Devil's claw – Wild yam – Wintergreen

ASTHMA
Black cohosh – Caffeine – Cranberry – Fenugreek – Lobelia capsules – Thyme

B

BEDWETTING
Bach's Rescue Remedy – Bach's Rock Water – Cream of Tartar – Cornsilk – Damiana

BLADDER INFECTIONS
Cornsilk – Cranberry juice – Echinacea – Juniper – Marsh mallow – Yarrow

BLOOD PRESSURE (HIGH)
Garlic – Hawthorn – Kava Kava – Kelp – Mistletoe – Yarrow

BLOOD PRESSURE (LOW)
Goldenseal – Ginger – Garlic – Siberian – Ginseng – Vitamin A – Vitamin B complex

BREAST-FEEDING (PROBLEMS PRODUCING)
Blessed thistle – Caraway seeds – Damiana – Fennel – Marsh mallow – Raspberry

BRUISES
Cider vinegar – Lavender – Hyssop – Oatmeal – Marigold oil – Vitamin E oil

BURNS
Aloe Vera – Camomile – Cucumber – Marigold – St John's Wort – Thyme

C

CANDIDA
Cabbage – Cranberry – Echinacea – Garlic – Tea Tree suppositories – Kava Kava

CATARRH
Echinacea – Fenugreek – Garlic – Goldenseal –

Olbus oil inhalant –
Peppermint

CHILBLAINS
Ginger – Horsetail – Red
pepper (cayenne powder)

CIRCULATION
– Garlic – Ginger –
Hawthorn – Horsetail
– Red pepper (cayenne
powder) – Rosemary

COLD, THE
Echinacea – Eucalyptus –
Garlic – Ginger –
Goldenseal – Vitamin C

COLIC
Angelica – Fennel – Ginger
– Juniper – Soya milk –
Valerian

CONJUNCTIVITIS
Bilberry – Camomile –
Eyebright – Fennel –
Goldenseal – Marigold

CONSTIPATION
Aloe Vera – Damiana –
Physalis fruit –
Psyllium – Rhubarb –
Senna

COUGH
Angelica – Aniseed –
Comfrey – Garlic –
Fenugreek – Goldenseal
Black cohosh –
Calendula – Evening
primrose capsules –
Feverfew – Runny
honey – Vitamin B6

DANDRUFF
Parsley – Sage – Stinging
nettle – Vitamin A –
Vitamin B6 – Zinc
DEPRESSION
Ginseng – Potassium –

Rosemary – St John's
Wort – Valerian –
Vitamin C

DERMATITIS
Aloe Vera – Comfrey –
Evening primrose –
Goldenseal – Vitamin
A – Vitamin B6

DIARRHOEA
Blessed thistle – Bilberry –
Comfrey – Folic acid –
Meadowsweet –
Vitamin A

DIVERTICULITIS
Camomile – Caraway seeds
– Comfrey – Fennel –
Psyllium – Wild yam

E

EARACHE
Calcium – Echinacea –
Garlic – St John's Wort
– Vitamin B complex –
Zinc

ECZEMA
Aloe Vera – Comfrey –
Goldenseal – Pansy –
Sulphur ointment –
Zinc ointment

F

FAINTING
Bach's Rescue Remedy –
Cup of coffee –
Lavender – Peppermint
– Valerian

FATIGUE
Damiana – Feverfew –
Gingko biloba –
Ginseng – St John's
Wort – Valerian
FEVER
Black cohosh – Calendula

– Ginger – Goldenseal
– Lobelia – Willow

FIBROSITIS
Echinacea – Ginger – Red
pepper (cayenne pow-
der) – St John's Wort –
Wintergreen

FLATULENCE
Angelica – Blessed thistle –
Caraway – Parsley –
Red pepper (cayenne
powder) – Valerian

FLU (INFLUENZA)
Blessed thistle – Calendula
– Echinacea –
Eucalyptus – Garlic –
Goldenseal – Myrrh

FOOD POISONING
Camomile – Dandelion tea
– Folic acid – Ginger –
Vitamin C – Vitamin E

FRECKLES
Cranberry juice –
Elderflower –
Horseradish –
Raspberry

FUNGAL INFECTIONS
Echinacea – Fenugreek –
Goldenseal – Marigold
– Myrrh – Tea tree oil

G

GINGIVITIS
Almond oil – Bilberry –
Echinacea – Elderberry
– Goldenseal – Green
tea

GOUT
Burdock – Calcium –
Dandelion – Lobelia –
Vitamin A – Vitamin E

GLANDS (SWOLLEN)
Red pepper (cayenne)

tincture – Echinacea –
Garlic – Lemon juice –
Marigold – Vitamin C

GLAUCOMA
Bilberry – Eyebright –
Vitamin A – Vitamin B
complex – Vitamin C –
Vitamin D

HAEMORRHOIDS
Comfrey – Dandelion –
Goldenseal – Lobelia –
Vitamin C – Vitamin B6

HALITOSIS
Dill – Fennel – Parsley –
Vitamin B6 – Vitamin
C – Zinc

HANGOVER
Feverfew – Onion soup –
Peppermint tea –
Porridge – Rosemary –
St John's Wort

HAYFEVER
Echinacea – Eyebright –
Goldenseal – Vitamin
B complex – Vitamin C
– Yarrow

HEADACHE
Calcium – Camomile –
Feverfew – St John's
Wort – Vitamin D –
Zinc

HEARTBURN
Camomile – Comfrey –
Ginger – Marsh mallow
– Meadowsweet –
Peppermint

**HORMONES (REGULATE AND
BALANCE)**
Damiana – Evening prim-
rose oil – Ginseng – St
John's Wort – Vitamin
B6 – Vitamin B12

I

IMMUNE SYSTEM
Echinacea – Gingko biloba
– Goldenseal – Korean
Ginseng – Vitamin B12
– Vitamin C

IMPOTENCE
Calcium – Damiana – Folic
acid – Iodine – Vitamin
E – Zinc

INDIGESTION
Blessed thistle – Camomile
– Fennel – Ginger –
Peppermint – Wild
yam

INFECTION
Echinacea – Garlic –
Goldenseal – Lobelia –
Uva Ursi – Vitamin C

INFLAMMATION
Aloe Vera – Black cohosh –
Burdock – Devil's claw
– Fenugreek – Ginger

INSOMNIA
California poppy –
Camomile – Damiana
– Hops – Lavender –
Valerian

ITCHING
Calendula – Camomile –
Cucumber –
Goldenseal – Marigold
– St John's Wort

JAUNDICE
Burdock – Dandelion –
Goldenseal – Vitamin
A – Vitamin B complex
– Wild yam

KIDNEYS
Bilberry – Dandelion –
Devil's claw – Garlic –
Vitamin A – Vitamin B
complex

L

LACTATION
Blessed thistle – Caraway –
Damiana – Fennel –
Marsh mallow –
Vitamin B6

LARYNGITIS
Caraway – Echinacea –
Fenugreek – Goldenseal
– Licorice – Red
pepper (cayenne
powder)

LIBIDO LOSS
Black cohosh – Camomile
– Damiana – Evening
primrose – Folic acid –
Valerian

LICE
Kwell – Pomegranate –
Powdered parsley –
Tansy – Tea tree oil –
Turmeric

LIVER
Bilberry – Burdock –
Dandelion –
Goldenseal – Vitamin
E – Wild yam

LOWER BACK PAIN
Calcium – Copper –
Devil's claw – Kelp –
Red pepper (cayenne
powder) – Wintergreen

M

MEMORY LOSS
Gingko biloba – Kelp – Korean Ginseng – Lobelia – Red pepper (cayenne powder) – Siberian Ginseng

MENOPAUSE
Black cohosh – Blessed thistle – Calcium – Goldenseal – Licorice – Siberian Ginseng

MENSTRUAL PROBLEMS
Blessed thistle – Calendula – Camomile – Iodine – Uva Ursi – Valerian

MIGRAINES
Calcium – Camomile – Feverfew – Magnesium – Potassium – Vitamin B3

MORNING SICKNESS
Camomile – Ginger – Raspberries – Peppermint – Vitamin C – Vitamin K

MOTION SICKNESS
Camomile – Charcoal tablets – Gingko biloba – Ginger – Meadowsweet – Vitamin B complex

MOUTH ULCERS
Aloe Vera – Goldenseal – Iron – Magnesium – Vitamin A – Zinc

MUMPS
Echinacea – Ginger – Lobelia – Vitamin A – Vitamin C – Vitamin E

N

NAUSEA
Ginger – Goldenseal – Magnesium – Meadowsweet – Peppermint – Red pepper (cayenne powder)

NEURALGIA
Black cohosh – Devil's claw – Echinacea – Goldenseal – St John's Wort – Valerian

NEURITIS
Black cohosh – Calcium – Devil's claw – Lobelia – Magnesium – Valerian

NOSEBLEEDS
Dandelion – Iron – Kelp – Magnesium – Potassium – Witch hazel

O

OBESITY
Fenugreek – Grapefruit oil – Hawthorn – Kelp – Licorice – Valerian

OEDEMA
Black cohosh – Blessed thistle – Cornsilk – Dandelion – Juniper – Uva Ursi

OSTEOARTHRITIS
Black cohosh – Burdock – Calcium – Devil's claw – Magnesium – Red pepper (cayenne powder)

OSTEOPOROSIS
Calcium – Copper – Devil's claw – Feverfew – Magnesium – Vitamin B12

P

PAIN
Black cohosh – Devil's claw – Kava Kava – Rosemary – Valerian – Willow

PALPITATIONS
Black cohosh – Damiana – Evening primrose oil – Lavender – St John's Wort – Valerian

PANIC ATTACKS
Black cohosh – Camomile – Damiana – Lavender – St John's Wort – Valerian

PLEURISY
Eucalyptus – Licorice – Lobelia – Nettle – Pleurisy root – Thyme

PNEUMONIA
Comfrey – Echinacea – Eucalyptus – Licorice – Vitamin A – Vitamin C

PREGNANCY
Folic acid – Ginger – Nettle tea – Magnesium – Meadowsweet – Peppermint

PRE-MENSTRUAL TENSION
Black cohosh – Blessed thistle – Calendula – Evening primrose oil – Lobelia – Valerian

PROSTATE
Cornsilk – Damiana – Kava Kava – Magnesium – Vitamin A – Zinc

PSORIASIS
Burdock – Dandelion – Goldenseal – Lobelia –

St John's Wort – Zinc
ointment

R

RHEUMATISM
Black cohosh – Calcium –
Camomile – Fennel –
Potassium – Zinc

S

SCIATICA
Black cohosh – Devil's claw
– St John's Wort –
Valerian – Vitamin D –
Vitamin E

SHINGLES
Calcium – Calendula –
Red pepper (cayenne)
cream – Magnesium –
Valerian – Wild yam

SINUSITIS
Black cohosh – Comfrey –
Eyebright – Fenugreek
– Goldenseal –
Potassium

SORE STOMACH
Damiana – Devil's claw –
Ginger – Meadowsweet
– Rosemary – Sage

SORE THROAT
Calendula – Devil's claw –
Echinacea – Garlic –
Hyssop – Marsh mal-
low

SPOTS
Aloe Vera juice – Echinacea
– Folic acid – Garlic –
Vitamin A – Vitamin B6

STIES
Beta-carotene – Bilberry –
Eyebright – Vitamin A

– Vitamin B complex –
Vitamin B6

STRESS
Bach's Rescue Remedy –
Damiana – Folic acid –
St John's Wort –
Valerian

STROKE
Comfrey – Evening primrose
oil – Goldenseal –
Vitamin B complex –
Vitamin B3 – Vitamin E

SUNBURN
Aloe Vera – Devil's claw –
Eyebright – Marigold –
St John's Wort –
Valerian

SWELLING
(*See* Oedema)

T

TEETHING
Aloe Vera gel – Cloves –
Lobelia gel –
Peppermint oil –
Thyme

TENSION
Bach's Rescue Remedy –
Camomile – Damiana
– St John's Wort –
Valerian

TINNITUS
Black cohosh – Calcium –
Gingko biloba –
Goldenseal –
Magnesium –
Potassium

TONSILLITIS
Devil's claw – Echinacea –
Garlic – Ginger –
Goldenseal – Myrrh

TOOTHACHE
Cloves – Devil's claw –

Goldenseal – Hops –
Thyme (gargle) –
Wintergreen

TRAVEL SICKNESS
Charcoal tablets –
Goldenseal –
Meadowsweet –
Peppermint – Valerian

U

ULCERS (EXTERNAL)
Comfrey – Echinacea –
Folic acid – Goldenseal
– Myrrh – Vitamin E

ULCERS (MOUTH)
(*See* Mouth ulcers)

ULCERS (STOMACH)
Comfrey – Echinacea –
Goldenseal – Licorice –
Meadowsweet –
Valerian

URINE INFECTION
Black cohosh – Cranberries
– Damiana –
Dandelion – Echinacea
– Goldenseal

V

VAGINAL INFECTION
Calendula – Cranberry –
Dandelion – Echinacea –
Tea tree oil – Vitamin C

VOMITING
Cloves – Comfrey –
Lavender – Marsh
malow – Meadowsweet
– Peppermint

WATER RETENTION
Burdock – Dandelion –
Juniper – Parsley – Uva
Ursi – Vitamin B6

WHOOPING COUGH
Black cohosh – Echinacea –
Garlic – Lobelia –
Pansy – Valerian

WOUNDS
Comfrey – Goldenseal –
Kelp – Marigold – Tea
tree – Vitamin K

Glossary of Herbal Remedies

A

ALMOND OIL
Abrasions – Cuts – Insect bites – Minor burns – Skin problems – Sunburn – Wounds

ALOE VERA
Abrasions – Cuts – Insect bites – Minor burns – Minor wounds – Skin problems – Sunburn –

ANGELICA
Colic – Heartburn – Indigestion – Menstrual cramps – Removes phlegm – Rheumatism – Skin lice – Tea can counteract cold – Upset stomach

ANISEED
Colds – Coughs – Increases milk in nursing women – Nausea

ASPIRIN
Fever – Headaches – Minor aches – Rheumatism – Stroke – Thinning blood

B

BACH'S RESCUE REMEDY
Anxiety – Bedwetting – Fainting – Irritability – Panic attacks

BASIL
Fever – Headaches – Indigestion – Induces menstruation – Nausea

BETA-CAROTENE
Psoriasis

BILBERRY
Angina – Diarrhoea – Conjunctivitis – Glaucoma – Lowers cholesterol – Liver problems – Menstrual cramps – Poor eyesight – Preserves eyesight – Sties – Stomach conditions

BLACKBERRY
Diarrhoea – Tonsillitis

BLACK COHOSH
As a relaxant – Arthritis – Asthma – Cramps – Fever – Helps lower blood pressure – Inflammation – Libido loss – Menopause – Most 'women's problems' – Neuralgia – Neuritis – PMT – Poisonous bites – Promotes labour and eases delivery – Relieves swelling – Rheumatism – Sciatica – Sinusitis

BLACK PEPPER
High blood pressure – Osteoporosis

BLESSED THISTLE
Appetite loss – Fever – Flatulence – Flu – Increases milk production – Indigestion – Liver problems – Menopause – Oedema – PMT – Regulates appetite – Regulates menstrual cycle

BUCHU
Bladder infections – Cystitis – Digestive disorders – Oedema – Water retention

BURDOCK
Acne – Allergies – canker sores – Cirrohosis of the liver – Dandruff – Disperses kidney stones – Diuretic – Eczema – Gout – Hives – Lowers blood sugar – Psoriasis – Slightly laxative – Stimulates liver – Wound healer

BUTCHER'S BROOM
Circulation – Diuretic –
Haemorrhoids –
Jaundice – Low blood
pressure – Relieving
oedema – Tinnitus –
Varicose veins

C

CABBAGE
Asthma – Morning sickness
– Ulcers

CAFFEINE
Asthma – Fainting

CALCIUM
Anxiety – Arthritis –
Backache – Bones –
Foot and leg cramps –
Growing pains –
Insomnia – Joint pains
– Menstrual cramps –
Nerves – PMT – Teeth

CALENDULA
Cramps – First-degree
burns – Flu – Itching –
PMT – Reducing fever
– Shingles – Sore throat
– Vaginal infections

CALIFORNIAN POPPY
Anxiety – Appetite loss –
Colic – Impotence –
Insomnia – Sedative for
kids – Tension

CAMOMILE
Anaemia – Anxiety – Back
pain – Boosts appetite
– Burns –
Conjunctivitis –
Diverticulitis – Food
poisoning – Headache
– Heartburn – Hysteria
– Indigestion –
Inflammation –
Insomnia – Itching –
Libido loss – Menstrual
problems – Migraine –
Morning/motion sick-
ness – Nausea – Nerves
– Nightmares – Panic
attacks – Rheumatism
– Skin irritations –
Wounds

CARAWAY
Colds – Coughs –
Digestion –
Diverticulitis – Infant
colic – Increases
appetite – Laryngitis –
Most stomach disorders
– Promotes breast milk

CARROT
Angina – Asthma –
Cataracts – Diarrhoea –
Liver problems – Skin
problems

CELERY
Arthritis – Diuretic – Gout
– Inflammation –
Rheumatism

CHARCOAL TABLETS
Nausea – Travel sickness

CIDER VINEGAR
Arthritis – Liver disorders –
Sunburn

CINNAMON
Erection problems – Fever
– Heartburn – Nausea

CLEAVERS
Abscesses – Acne –
Adenoids – Bladder
infections – Boils –
Cystitis – Eczema –
Itching – PMT –
Psoriasis – Tonsillitis

CLOVES
Antiseptic – Aphrodisiac –
Digestive system –
Flatulence – Mild anaes-
thetic – Teething –
Toothache – Vomiting

COMFREY
Bronchitis – Bruises –
Catarrh – Coughs –
Dandruff – Dermatitis
– Diarrhoea –
Diverticulitis – Eczema
– Good for broken
bones – Haemorrhoids
– Heartburn – Helps
'knit' skin wounds –
Sinusitis – Sore nipples
– Stomach ulcers –
Stroke – Ulcers –
Vomiting

COPPER
Assists development of
bones, brain, nerves
and skin – Digestive
system – Eyes – Slows
baldness

CORNSILK
Bedwetting – Bladder
infections – Cystitis –
Inflammation of
bladder/kidney/urethra
– Kidney stones –
Oedema – Prostate

CRANBERRY
Antibiotic – Anxiety –
Asthma – Candida –
Bladder infections –
Fever – Fights bacteria
– Oedema – Water
retention

D

DAMIANA
Depression – Impotence –
Laxative – Nerve tonic
– Panic attacks –
Urinary antiseptic

DANDELION
Alcoholism – Anaemia –
Blood cleanser –
Cirrhosis – Dermatitis
– Digestion – Gout –
Kidney stones – Liver

disorder – Loss of
appetite – Oedema –
Rheumatic fever –
Senility – Tumours –
Water retention

DEVIL'S CLAW
Arthritis – Blood purifier –
Gall bladder –
Indigestion –
Inflammation – Lowers
back pain – Loss of
appetite – Pain relief

DILL
Colic – Flatulence –
Halitosis – Heartburn –
Indigestion – Promotes
breast milk

ECHINACEA
Acne – Blood purifier –
Catarrh – Chronic
fatigue – Cirrhosis of
the liver – Colds –
Crohn's Disease –
Croup – Earache – Ear
infections – Flu –
Fungal infections –
Gingivitis – Hayfever –
Immune deficiency –
Minor infections –
Mumps – Pneumonia –
Swollen glands –
Tonsillitis – Warts

ELDERBERRY
Bronchitis – Colds – Fever
– Flu – Gingivitis

EUCALYPTUS
Asthma – Bronchitis –
Catarrh – Colds – Flu
– Pleurisy – Pneumonia

EYEBRIGHT
Allergies – Cataracts –
Conjunctivitis –
Glaucoma – Hayfever –
Night blindness –

Sinusitis – Sinus
problems – Sties –
Sunburn

F

FENNEL
Breast-feeding – Cirrhosis
of the liver – Colic –
Digestive problems –
Diverticulitis –
Indigestion – Lactation

FENUGREEK
Anaemia – Asthma –
Croup – Fever – Flu –
Fungal infections –
Gastro-intestinal
irritation – Indigestion
– Inflammation –
Laryngitis – Pneumonia
– Rheumatics

FEVERFEW
Cramps – Headaches –
Migraine –
Osteoporosis

FOLIC ACID
Diarrhoea – Food poison-
ing – Impotence –
Libido loss – Spots –
Stress – Ulcers (N.B.
Advisable to take prior
to pregnancy if plan-
ning, as reports suggest
a significant decrease in
foetus having Spina
Bifida)

G

GARLIC
Abscesses – Acne –
Adenoids – Candida –
Colds – Cough –
Earache – Flu – High
blood pressure –
Kidneys – Sore throat –
Swollen glands –

Tonsillitis – Whooping
cough

GINGER
Chilblains – Colds – Colic
– Digestive problems –
Fibrositis – Flatulence –
Food poisoning –
Heartburn – Morning
sickness – Motion sick-
ness – Mumps –
Nausea – Sore stomach
– Tonsillitis

GINGKO BILOBA
Circulation – Fatigue –
Immune system – Leg
ulcers – Memory loss –
Motion sickness –
Phlebitis – Senility

GINSENG (AMERICAN)
Athletic performance –
Energy – Fatigue –
Gastro-intestinal prob-
lems – Infection –
Stress
(*See also* Korean ginseng)

GINSENG (SIBERIAN)
Colds – Diabetes – Flu –
Memory
(*See also* Korean ginseng)

GOLDENSEAL
Abscesses – Adenoids –
Alcoholism – Appetite
loss – Blood clots –
Bowel cleanser –
Catarrh –
Conjunctivitis – Cough
– Dermatitis – Eczema
– Fever – Flu –
Gingivitis –
Haemorrhoids –
Infections – Immune
system – Itching –
Jaundice – Liver
disorders – Menopause
– Mouth ulcers –
Nausea – Psoriasis –
Sinusitis – Stroke –
Tinnitus – Tonsillitis –
Toothache – Travel

sickness – Ulcers –
Urine infections –
Wounds

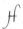

HAWTHORN
Angina – Blood pressure –
Circulation –
Congestive heart failure
– Obesity – Varicose
veins

HONEY
Cough – Hangover –
Wounds

HONEYSUCKLE
Bronchitis – Colds –
Earache – Flu – Sore
throat – Tonsillitis

HOPS
Insomnia – Toothache

HORSETAIL
Circulation – Flatulence –
Leg cramps –
Osteoporosis

HYSSOP
Blood pressure – Bruises –
Epilepsy – Sore throat

I

IODINE
Boils – Corns – Cuts –
Sunburn

IPRIFLAVONE
Osteoporosis

IVY
Bronchitis – Laryngitis –
Skin problems – Yeast
infections

J

JASMINE
Breast-feeding problems

JAVA TEA
Kidney stones

JUNIPER
Viral infections – Water
retention

K

KAVA KAVA
Anxiety – Blood pressure –
Candida – Fluid
retention – Insomnia –
Nervousness – Over-
eating – Pain – Prostate
– Stress

KELP
Anaemia – Circulation –
Cold feet – Dieting –
Energy – Fluid
retention – Goitre –
Hair – High blood
pressure – Lower back
pain – Memory loss –
Nails – Nosebleeds –
Obesity – Thyroid
gland – Wounds

KOREAN GINSENG
(Same as Asian and
Chinese)
Cholesterol – Circulation –
Concentration –
Depression –
Exhaustion – Fatigue –
Immune system –
Memory – Menopause
– Recuperation –
Regulates hormones
(Do not use with Vitamin C)

KWELL
Lice

L

LAVENDER
Altitude sickness –
Depression – Digestive
system – Exhaustion –
Fainting – Flatulence –
Headaches – Neuralgia
– Palpitations – Panic
attacks – Rheumatism
– Sleeping aid – Stress
– Relaxant – Vomiting

LICORICE
Arthritis – Asthma –
Catarrh – Cleans teeth
– Colds – Colic –
Congestion – Dry
cough – Flu –
Laryngitis – Lung dis-
orders – Menopause –
Obesity – Pneumonia –
Prevents tooth decay –
Sore throat – Stiffness –
Stomach ulcers – Stress

LOBELIA
Asthma – Bronchitis –
Catarrh – Earache –
Fever – Gout –
Haemorrhoids – Helps
stop smoking –
Infection – Memory
loss – Neuritis –
Pleurisy – PMT –
Pneumonia – Psoriasis
– Reduces heart
palpitations – Teething
– Whooping cough

M

MAGNESIUM
Alcoholism – Allergies –
Anti-stress – Baldness –
Cataracts – Circulation
– Constipation –
Cystitis – Depression –
Diarrhoea – Eczema –
Fatigue – Gout –
Halitosis – Headache –

Helps prevent heart disease – High blood pressure – Indigestion – Insomnia – Kidney stones – Leg cramps – Leg ulcers – Lowers cholesterol – Menopause – Migraines – Mouth sores – Nervousness – Neuritis – Obesity – Osteoarthritis – Osteoporosis – Prevents blood clots – Prostate – Rheumatism – Shingles – Stomach acid – Tinnitus – Tooth decay

MARIGOLD

Adenoids – Bruises – Burns – Conjunctivitis – Fungal infections – Itching – Sunburn – Swollen glands – Wounds

MARSH MALLOW

Abscesses – Bladder infections – Breast-feeding – Breathing problems – Bronchitis – Bruises – Burns – Colds – Congestion – Cystitis – Expectorant – Flu – Heartburn – Indigestion – Lactation – Pains – Sore throat – Upset stomach – Whooping cough

MEADOWSWEET

Diarrhoea – Heartburn – Morning sickness – Motion sickness – Nausea – Sore/upset stomach – Stomach ulcer – Vomiting

MILK THISTLE

Eczema – Liver disorders – Pollution – Psoriasis

MISTLETOE

High blood pressure

MYRRH

Abscesses – Appetite builder – Fever – Flu – Fungal infections – Gum disease – Halitosis – Lung disease – Tonsillitis – Skin ulcers – Stomach ulcers

N

NETTLE

Alcoholism – Allergies – Asthma – Baldness – Dandruff – Epilepsy – Hayfever – Pleurisy

NETTLE JUICE

Anaemia

O

ONION

Allergies – Asthma – Burns – Colds – Insect bites – Pneumonia – Scabies

OREGANO

Arthritis – Asthma – Sinusitis

P

PANSY

Whooping cough

PARSLEY

Diuretic – Flatulence – Kidney stones – Lice – Oedema – Water retention

PEPPERMINT

Altitude sickness – Catarrh – Colic – Colitis – Congestion – Fainting – Flatulence – Halitosis

– Heartburn – Indigestion – Morning sickness – Nausea – Teething – Travel sickness – Vomiting

PHYLUM

Bowel cleanser – Constipation – Diverticulitis – Haemorrhoids

PHYSALIS FRUIT

Bowel cleansing – Constipation

PLEURISY ROOT

Pleurisy

POTASSIUM

Flatulence – Halitosis – Migraines – Nose bleeds – Rheumatism – Tinnitus

Q

QUERCETIN

Asthma – Itching – Scabies – Skin problems

R

RASPBERRY

Bowel cleanser – Breast-feeding – Freckles – Menstrual problems – Morning sickness – Mouth sores – Nausea – Stomach ulcers

RED CLOVES

Acne – Chickenpox – Cirrhosis of the liver – Hiatus hernia – Menopausal difficulties – Nausea – Rheumatism

RED PEPPER (cayenne

powder)

Chilblains – Circulation – Cold feet – Fibrositis – Flatulence – Inflammation – Memory – Nausea – Shingles

RHUBARB
Constipation

RIBOFLAVIN
(*See* Vitamin B2)

ROSE HIPS
Colds – Flu – Heart attack – Nausea – Stroke

ROSEMARY
Baldness – Circulation – Halitosis – Hangover – Lack of appetite – Memory – Pain – Sore stomach

RUNNY HONEY
Cramps

S

SKULLCAP
Alcoholism – Anxiety – Athletic injuries – Depression – Ear infections – Epilepsy – Hyperactivity – Insomnia – Leg cramps – Nervous problems – Neuritis – PMT – Psoriasis – Smoking – Stress – Tension

U

UVA URSI
Diabetes – Infection – Kidney stones – Menstrual problems – Oedema – Water retention

V

VALERIAN
Alcoholism – Anxiety – Colic – Colitis – Depression – Fainting – Flatulence – High blood pressure – Hyperactivity – Insomnia – Menstrual problems – Nervous problems – Neuralgia – Neuritis – Obesity – Pain – Palpitations – Panic attacks – PMT – Sciatica – Shingles – Smoking – Stomach ulcers – Stress – Sunburn – Teeth grinding – Tension – Travel sickness – Whooping cough

VITAMIN A
Acne – Alcoholism – Allergies – Asthma – Baldness – Boils – Bronchitis – Bursitis – Canker sores – Chickenpox – Chronic fatigue – Circulation – Cirrhosis of the liver – Colds and flu – Colitis – Constipation – Coughs – Croup – Cystitis – Dandruff – Dermatitis – Diabetes – Diarrhoea – Digestive problems – Ear infections – Eczema – Eye problems – Fever – Glaucoma – Gout – Goitre – Haemorrhoids – Halitosis – Hayfever – Headache – Hiatus hernia – High and low blood pressure – Immune deficiency – Infertility – Jaundice – Kidney stones – Leg ulcers – Liver disorders – Menopause – Mouth sores – Mumps – Pneumonia – Pre-natal preparation – Psoriasis – Senility – Shingles – Sinus problems – Spots – Stomach ulcers – Stress – Tinnitus – Yeast infections – Warts – Whooping cough

VITAMIN B COMPLEX
Acne – Alcoholism – Allergies – Arthritis – Asthma – Baldness – Blood clots – Bowel cleanser – Colitis – Constipation – Cystitis – Dandruff – Dermatitis – Diabetes – Digestive problems – Drug addictions – Ear infections – Eczema – Emphysema – Epilepsy – Fevers and flu – Flatulence – Glaucoma – Goitre – Gout – Haemorrhoids – Halitosis – Hayfever – Headache – Heart attack – Hiatus hernia – High and low blood pressure – Hyperthyroidism – Hypoglycaemia – Infertility – Insomnia – Jet lag – Kidney stones – Leg cramps – Liver disorders – Menopause – Menstrual problems – Migraines – Motion sickness – Mouth sores – Mumps – Muscular dystrophy – Nervous problems – Neuritis – Obesity – Oedema – Osteoarthritis – Pneumonia – Pre-natal preparation – Psoriasis – Rheumatism – Sciatica – Senility – Shingles – Sinus problems – Stress – Stomach ulcers – Stroke – Sunburn – Tinnitus –

Tumours – Varicose veins – Warts – Whooping cough

VITAMIN B2

Asthma – Cataracts – Dermatitis – Diabetes – Diarrhoea – Eye problems – Glaucoma

VITAMIN B3

Acne – Allergies – Arthritis – Asthma – Baldness – Blood clots – Circulation – Cirrhosis of the liver – Dermatitis – Digestive problems – Eye problems – Fevers and flu – Halitosis – High blood pressure – Migraines – Stroke

VITAMIN B5

Allergies – Asthma – Canker sores – High blood pressure – Low blood pressure

VITAMIN B6

Acne – Allergies – Asthma – Colds and flu – Colitis – Coughs – Dandruff – Depression – Dermatitis – Diabetes – Diarrhoea – Epilepsy – Eye problems – Goitre – Halitosis – Immune deficiency – Morning sickness – Oedema – Water retention

VITAMIN B12

Allergies – Asthma – Bronchitis – Bursitis – Canker sores – Cirrhosis of the liver – Depression – Diabetes – Immune deficiency – Leg ulcers – Osteoporosis

VITAMIN C

Acne – Alcoholism – Allergies – Anaemia – Arthritis – Asthma – Bee stings – Blood clots – Boils – Breast-feeding – Breathing problems – Bronchitis – Burns – Bursitis – Canker sores – Chickenpox – Chronic fatigue – Circulation – Cirrhosis of the liver – Colds and flu – Colitis – Constipation – Coughs – Croup – Dandruff – Depression – Dermatitis – Diabetes – Diarrhoea – Digestive problems – Drug addictions – Ear infections – Eczema – Emphysema – Epilepsy – Eye problems – Fevers and flu – Food poisoning – Glaucoma – Goitre – Gout – Hayfever – Headaches – Haemorrhoids – Hiatus hernia – Hyperactivity – Hyperglycaemia – Hyperthyroidism – Hypothyroidism – Immune deficiency – Jet lag – Kidney stones – Leg cramps – Leg ulcers – Liver disorders – Melanoma – Menopause – Menstrual problems – Migraines – Mononucleosis – Morning sickness – Mouth sores – Mumps – Muscular dystrophy – Nausea – Nervous problems – Obesity – Oedema – Osteoarthritis – Osteoporosis – Pneumonia – Pre-natal preparation – Psoriasis – Rheumatism –

Senility – Shingles – Sinus problems – Smoking – Stress – Stroke – Sunburn – Tinnitus – Tumours – Skin ulcers – Stomach ulcers – Varicose veins – Warts – Water retention – Whooping cough – Yeast infection

VITAMIN D

Alcoholism – Arthritis – Chronic fatigue – Cirrhosis of the liver – Constipation – Cystitis – Dermatitis – Eczema – Emphysema – Epilepsy – Eye problems – Glaucoma – Headache – High and low blood pressure – Insomnia – Leg cramps – Menopause – Oedema – Osteoarthritis – Pre-natal preparation – Psoriasis – Sciatica – Shingles – Stress – Stomach ulcers

VITAMIN E

Acne – Alcoholism – Allergies – Arthritis – Asthma – Blood clots – Boils – Bronchitis – Burns – Bursitis – Chickenpox – Chronic fatigue – Circulation – Cirrhosis of the liver – Cold feet – Cold sores – Colitis – Constipation – Crohn's disease – Croup – Cystitis – Dandruff – Dermatitis – Diabetes – Emphysema – Epilepsy – Eye problems – Fevers and flu – Food poisoning – Glaucoma – Goitre – Gout – Hayfever – Haemorrhoids – High and low blood pressure

– Immune deficiency –
Infertility – Jet lag –
Kidney stones – Leg
cramps – Liver
disorders – Menopause
– Mouth sores –
Mumps – Muscular
dystrophy – Nervous
problems – Obesity –
Oedema –
Osteoarthritis –
Osteoporosis –
Osteoarthritis –
Pneumonia – Psoriasis
– Rheumatism –
Senility – Sinus
problems – Skin ulcers
– Stress – Stomach
ulcers – Stroke –
Sunburn – Tinnitus –
Tumours – Varicose
veins – Warts – Yeast
infection

VITAMIN F

Acne – Allergies – Arthritis
– Asthma

VITAMIN, MULTI

Anaemia – Athletic injuries
– Chickenpox –
Immune deficiency –
Night blindness –
Rheumatic fever –
Smoking – Tonsillitis
(N.B. Multi-vitamins are
good on the whole but if
you are lacking one specific
vitamin, you may find

multi-vitamins don't
contain enough of what
you need!)

VITAMIN, 'PABA'

Asthma – Burns – Halitosis
– Impotence –
Migraine

W

WILD YAM

Arthritis – Colitis –
Diverticulitis – Gastro-
intestinal irritation –
Indigestion – Jaundice
– Liver disorders –
Shingles

WILLOW

Fever – Pain

WINTERGREEN

Arthritis – Fibrositis –
Lower back pain –
Toothache

WITCH HAZEL

Acne – Diarrhoea –
Haemorrhoids – Nose
bleeds – Varicose veins

Y

YARROW

Bladder infections –
Circulation – Dandruff
– Hayfever – High
blood pressure – Leg
ulcers – Oedema –
Phlebitis – Tinnitus –
Varicose veins

YELLOW DOCK

Acne – Anaemia – Baldness
– Blood purifier –
Dermatitis – Eczema –
Haemorrhoids –
Senility

YUCCA

Aches and pains – Arthritis
– Baldness –
Depression – Diarrhoea
– Gout – Obesity –
Oedema – Rheumatism

Z

ZINC

Constipation – Dandruff –
Earache – Halitosis –
Headache – Impotence
– Rheumatism –
Varicose veins

Index